HEALTHY EATING:
FACT AND FICTION

HEALTHY EATING: FACT AND FICTION

Edited by Anna Bradley

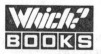

Published by Consumers' Association
and Hodder & Stoughton

Which? Books are commissioned and researched by
The Association for Consumer Research
and published by Consumers' Association,
2 Marylebone Road, London NW1 4DX
and Hodder & Stoughton, 47 Bedford Square,
London WC1B 3DP

British Library Cataloguing in Publication Data
Healthy eating.
  1. Man. Health. Effects of diet
  I. Bradley, Anna
  613.2

ISBN 0 340 488 75-1

Typographic design by Paul Saunders
Cover illustration by John Holder

Typeset by Litho Link Limited, Welshpool, Wales
Printed and bound in Great Britain by BPCC Hazell Books Ltd
Member of BPCC Ltd, Aylesbury, Bucks, England

CONTENTS

HEALTHY EATING –

WHAT IS IT?

Over the past decade or so, the media have been giving out a bewildering stream of often contradictory messages about what we should eat for the sake of our health. No sooner, it seemed, had Audrey Eyton's F-Plan diet book brought attention to the virtues of eating more fibre, than there were warnings of 'muesli-belt malnutrition' – children being denied essential nutrients by the faddy regimes of their parents. At the same time, slowly but surely, fat and cholesterol were coming to be seen as out-and-out villains, causes of heart disease. The dairy industry retaliated with a nostalgic advertising campaign urging us to return to the 'traditional' taste of butter. And the view that fruit may be as bad for your teeth as chocolate has emerged to challenge conventional wisdom of eating an apple a day.

Why is there so much confusion over what we should eat? Why do food manufacturers say there is no proof that the British diet is harmful to health, while the supermarkets are busy producing leaflets telling customers how to change their eating patterns for the better? Why do a few experts disagree vehemently on the health risks of various types of food?

This book aims to unravel the tangled threads of the arguments about food and health, so that you can decide for yourself whether you want to change what you eat. It explains which assertions scientists, doctors, nutritionists and dietitians are agreed on, but also points out where they differ in their interpretation of food and health studies. Also explained is why, in many cases, the evidence linking particular aspects of diet and health falls short of concrete proof.

A key to deciding whether you want to change your diet is to find out exactly what you do eat. Many reports and recommendations on a healthy diet are based on the so-called 'average' diet, to which very few, if any, of us actually conform. To help you find out the implications of your eating pattern, *Which?* has devised, with the Nuffield Laboratories for Comparative Medicine, a questionnaire (see page 127) about intakes of five nutrients – fat, saturated fat, fibre, salt and sugar. If, having filled it in, you opt to make some changes to what you consume, you can always come back and fill it in again some months later – there are duplicate copies at the end of the book.

This is a book about diet in the broadest sense – what we actually consume over a period of time. It is not about dieting or losing weight. Nor will it dogmatically tell you what you should be eating for your health.

The links between food and health

1
THE DEBATE SO FAR

Now that the killer diseases of the eighteenth and nineteenth centuries have been eradicated, it seems that one of the greatest threats to health may be the way we live. It is estimated that between 75 and 90 per cent of cancers, for example, could be prevented by our improving our environment and lifestyle – stopping smoking, changing drinking and eating habits and reducing pollution, among other things. In the late 1970s two leading cancer experts, Doll and Peto, examined all the evidence that had been collected about the causes of what are believed to be preventable cancers. They concluded that diet plays some part in the development of about one in three of such cases. (The estimates in the studies they reviewed varied from one in ten cancers being related to diet to seven in ten.) By contrast, they concluded that those perceived villains of our time, food additives, played a part in no more than one in a hundred cases of preventable cancer. (Doll and Peto, *The Causes of Cancer*, OUP, 1981.)

Adverse reactions like asthma, eczema or migraine are also more likely to be caused by the nature of particular foods than by food additives. Recent attempts by the Ministry of Agriculture, Fisheries and Food (MAFF) to assess the prevalence of adverse reactions to certain items, for instance milk and strawberries and to food additives, have concluded that 1 to 2.6 in 10,000 people are likely to be affected by food additives, but that 30 times as many, that is 30 to 85 in 10,000 people, are thought likely to be affected by some sort of food.

These are just two of the ways in which the sorts of food we choose to eat – as opposed to the quality of individual items – is thought to affect our health. The most widely publicised possible long-term links, though, are between fat and heart disease, sugar and tooth decay, and salt and high blood pressure. It has also been suggested that diet may play some part in causing diseases and disorders such as diabetes, gallstones, constipation and other bowel complaints, and may play a part in arthritis.

Two reports – broadly similar conclusions

Attention has been focused on the relationship between our health and what we eat since two reports were published with much media fanfare: the National Advisory Committee on Nutrition Education (NACNE) report, prepared by the then Health Education Council and the British Nutrition Foundation, published in 1983, and the Committee on Medical Aspects of Food Policy (COMA) report on *Diet and Cardiovascular Disease*, published a year later, in 1984, by the Department of Health (then part of the DHSS). While the COMA report was specifically about heart disease, NACNE's was called *A Discussion Paper on Proposals for Nutritional Guidelines for Health Education in Britain*, which aimed to give a wider view on what constitutes a healthy diet. Both reports found that the average British diet is high in fat, low in fibre and higher in sugar and salt than it need be. Both reports said that this sort of diet predisposes people to develop certain diseases, and concluded that the incidence of these diseases could be reduced if the average diet were changed in various ways (see Table 1).

If that sounds cautious, it's not surprising; the committees, especially COMA, chose their words extremely carefully. A complicating factor is that the 'average' diet is eaten by probably very few people, if any at all, since it is derived from figures for food sales and surveys of what people say they eat, as opposed to what they truly eat, and takes into account vegans and vegetarians at one end of the spectrum and chip addicts at the other. This makes it difficult to assess how far the recommendations apply to individuals. To be fair, NACNE and COMA were not attempting to point individuals to a route to

Table 1: The NACNE and COMA recommendations for the composition of a healthy diet

The 1983 NACNE report contained two sets of recommendations: one that could be achieved in the five to seven years following the publication of the report, and a longer-term plan to be achieved in 15 years from its publication.

Nutrient	COMA	NACNE-short term	NACNE-long term	Current average intake (1986)
Total fat	35% of total Calories	34% of total Calories	30% of total Calories	42.6% of total Calories
Saturated fat	15% of total Calories	15% of total Calories	10% of total Calories	15.9% of total Calories
Polyunsaturated fat	No specific recommendation	5% of total Calories	5% of total Calories minimum	5.5% of total Calories
Fibre	25 grams a day	25 grams a day	30 grams a day	20 grams a day
Sugar	Current intakes should not be increased	Reduce intakes by 10% (to 34 kilos a year)	Reduce by a further 40% (to 20 kilos a year)	38 kilos a year
Salt	Current intakes should not be increased and a decrease should be considered	Reduce intakes by 10% (to about 9 grams a day)	Reduce by a further (to about 7 grams a day)	10 grams a day

longer life; their purpose was to establish a path for national health campaigns.

Another important point is that when a report says that reductions in the average intake of fat would lead to a reduction in the incidence of heart disease, you cannot conclude that if you reduced your fat intake you would necessarily lower your risk of getting heart disease. Your fat intake may already be below average levels, or you may have an exceptionally high, or low, risks of developing heart disease for other reasons altogether – your smoking habits or your family history, for example.

The publication of the NACNE report in 1983 followed an acrimonious debate in the media. The report was commissioned by NACNE to provide it with an authoritative statement of the present consensus among experts as to what constitutes a healthy diet, which it felt it needed before it could embark on the task set by the Government of furthering nutrition education in Britain.

NACNE was made up of representatives from the Department of Health (then part of the DHSS), MAFF, the British Nutrition Foundation (BNF), a food-industry-funded research body, and the Health Education Council (HEC), now Authority, and a number of independent experts. When this ad hoc committee attempted a first draft of the report in 1981, its members couldn't agree on what to say. It took two years, four drafts and a bitter public debate for the report to be published, and then with the status only of a discussion document, for distribution to nutrition educators.

Given that it had so little official standing, the NACNE report has had surprising impact; it is widely quoted in academic and popular articles and is used by many nutritionists as the basis for their advice. This is because it is the only report which has attempted to give a clear statement of the consensus among experts on all aspects to diet and then gone on to make quantified recommendations about the changes that need to be made in the average diet. NACNE doesn't just say it is desirable to eat less fat, for example, it says how much less fat.

The COMA report has a quite different standing, partly because COMA advises the Government, partly because it was produced at the direct request of the DHSS. The panel was briefed to look only at the links between diet and cardiovascular disease – disease of the heart and blood vessels – and consequently their recommendations are more limited than those of the NACNE panel. The COMA report concentrates on fat and especially saturated fat, but the report does make some comments about other aspects of diet, in particular the need to ensure a balance in the diet when making some changes in it. The Government has since accepted the COMA report and thus has committed itself to implementing its recommendations, including some on the labelling of fat in food.

The picture worldwide

Individual scientists have been pointing to links between aspects of diet and certain diseases since the beginning of the century, and over the past 20 years or so there has been a stream of reports on diet from scientific bodies. In Scandinavia, expert committees recommended dietary changes as early as 1968; by 1975 reports had been published in New Zealand, the USA, the Netherlands, Australia and West Germany; by 1980 reports had been published in Canada and by the World Health Organisation, and there were further reports in Australia and the USA.

The vast majority of these expert committees have found that some sort of change to the western diet is desirable. Some reports cover a great deal of ground, some concentrate on one aspect of diet, or one sort of disease, and some conclude that the evidence is stronger in some areas than others and so limit their recommendations, but in general, they are in agreement. In *The Politics of Food* (Century Hutchinson, 1987) Geoffrey Cannon analysed 65 official reports produced between 1965 and 1985 and concluded that of these, no fewer than 59 recommended that at least some people should reduce fat intakes, and 55 of them singled out saturated fats; 50 of the reports recommended that less sugar should be eaten; 33 recommended more fibre and 36 less salt.

Take, for example, the first statement of dietary goals in the USA in 1977. It recommended that Americans should:

- reduce total fat by 25 per cent
- reduce saturated fat by 40 per cent
- reduce sugar intake by 40 per cent
- reduce salt intake by at least 50 per cent.

Despite the weight of international expert opinion, it took the publication of NACNE and COMA to generate discussion in Britain of dietary change. For the first time the views expressed in these two reports were supported by the majority of British experts, who now think that in general, the health of the British people would benefit if, on average, we ate more fibre and less fat, sugar and salt.

However, there is still a significant minority of scientists who are not persuaded, saying that the case for dietary change is not proven. Some even believe that it is irresponsible to advise people to change their diet when we can't be sure that changes would be beneficial. So, how is it that, even in the light of persuasive reports, experts with the same sort of training can disagree so vehemently about whether or not we should be changing what we eat?

Why different experts give different advice . . .

The fact is that both sets of experts are right: the bulk of the evidence supports the theory that certain aspects of diet are related to the incidence of certain diseases, and that changing the diet in appropriate ways will reduce the incidence of these diseases. But on the other hand, the evidence falls short of proof, and it is proof, or certainty, that the scientific cynics want before they firmly recommend people to change their diet.

Proof is what scientists are trained to demand. The causes of the killer diseases of the nineteenth and early twentieth centuries – tuberculosis, smallpox, typhoid and cholera – have all been traced. Although you were more likely to become infected if you lived in certain conditions, ultimately you would catch each of these diseases only if you came into contact with a particular virus or bacillus. This meant that people could be protected from it, or treated if they caught it; the disease could be cured. Scientists did not always understand the causes of the diseases when they first learnt how to protect people from them, but eventually they learnt exactly how and why they developed.

The major killer diseases of today – for example coronary heart disease and cancer – are far more complex: they appear not to have any simple, single external cause and they are not generally infectious; instead they are what is called 'multifactorial' – many factors affect an individual's chances of getting the disease – and instead of being caused by a foreign organism (a virus or bacterium), they tend to be caused by some degeneration of our own body. All this makes it much more difficult for scientists to understand the diseases, how and why they develop and how to prevent them.

The effect of lifestyle

Experts are agreed that the major diseases of today are caused by environmental or lifestyle factors, such as occupation, diet, exercise, smoking, and alcohol consumption, and if the precise causes could be pin pointed, the diseases could be prevented. Patterns of disease vary in different countries and between groups of people within countries, and sometimes lifestyles and habits vary between the same group of people, suggesting that there may be some sort of link between the disease and the lifestyle.

Take the five diseases most widely thought to be related to diet: coronary heart disease (CHD), cancer of the bowel and breast, cerebrovascular disease (stroke and high blood pressure) and stomach cancer. While CHD and cancers of the bowel and breast are common in the west and have a low incidence in Japan, cancer of the stomach and cerebrovascular disease are common in Japan and relatively low in incidence in America.

Moreover, studies have shown that if a group of people from a community exhibiting one sort of disease pattern moves into a community with a different disease incidence, in time, the immigrants may develop the disease patterns of their host community. American-born children of Japanese immigrants have quite a different pattern of disease from their parents: the incidence of CHD and breast and bowel cancer increase and that of stomach cancer and cerebrovascular disease falls. By the second generation, Japanese Americans have the same patterns of disease as their compatriots.

Since, in such instances, the genetic make-up of these people has not changed, the cause of the changed disease patterns must be sought in aspects of the environment or lifestyle which have changed – the amount of pollution in the air, eating habits, new sorts of working conditions and so on. But determining exactly which aspects of the environment may be involved in the development of a disease is very difficult.

The majority of the evidence is epidemiological, that is, put together by comparing groups of people and their lifestyles to see what possible explanations there might be for any differences in disease incidence between the two groups, as in the Japanese example above. Epidemiology can involve comparing the populations of different countries, people in different parts of the same country, different groups of people (for example some with high blood pressure and some with normal blood pressure), the same people moving from one country to another, or the same, or similar groups of people at different times (for example this year and ten years ago).

Comparisons like the Japanese one above give us clues but not proof – it may be that the major environmental difference between Japanese and American lifestyles is diet, but it may be some other factor. Also, links between disease and environment are rarely simple; it is normal for more than one factor to be associated with a disease. Incidence of heart disease, for example, shows a strong correlation not just with fat intakes, but also with television and home computer ownership, car driving and the country's gross national product, all of which reflect the degree of westernisation of lifestyle.

A further shortcoming of epidemiology is that it relies on the comparison of statistics, which though available for developed countries, are patchy in the developing world. There may also be a lack of consensus about the diagnosis of a disease, so deaths may be attributed to some other cause, making it difficult to compare the figures for different countries.

Dietary statistics are also notoriously difficult to collect. Food consumption figures are available for only 20 countries and then for only about 60 food items. Even in countries like Britain, where a good range of figures is available, inaccuracies occur because of the way they are collected and analysed (see Chapter 2 for more about the collection of dietary data in the UK).

Pros and cons of dietary trials

Epidemiology is a very useful first step in finding the links between diet and disease but it will never be able to prove that food 'x', or an excess of nutrient 'y' causes, say, heart disease. Specific experiments or trials can take scientists a stage further, and three types are used: retrospective studies, which ask people about their past habits in relation to diseases they have already contracted; prospective studies, which monitor people's lifestyle and disease over an extended period of time; and intervention studies, which ask one group of people to change their habits, while a control group retains the old lifestyle.

Retrospective studies try to establish how a group of people with a disease have differed in their lifestyle from a group similar in every respect, except that they do not have the disease. The main problem here for an assessment of diet is that people have a very imperfect recollection of the type of food they were eating 10 or 20 years ago, so the information gathered cannot be considered as reliable.

Prospective studies, in which a very large group of people undergo an array of medical tests and checks at regular intervals, while their lifestyle and disease incidence are also monitored, are rare, because they are difficult to control and often fail to be conclusive. Many of the checks and analyses that are carried out may be quite fruitless.

Finally, intervention trials are prohibitively expensive and may also prove inconclusive. A five-year intervention study in the Finnish province of North Karelia in the 1970s showed that a community programme to encourage people to reduce their risk factors of CHD could work. The population of an entire province were encouraged to change their diet, reduce fat and especially saturated fat intakes, have all cases of high blood pressure identified and treated, and reduce cigarette smoking. The incidence of CHD (the highest in the world at the time) went down but, to confuse the picture, the incidence of CHD also fell in the neighbouring province, which was being used as a control, and where no specific dietary advice was being given. It may well be that people in the control province heard of the advice being given to their neighbours and started to take their own preventive action, but even if that is the explanation, doubt was thrown on what otherwise was a fairly conclusive study.

Another intervention trial, known as MRFIT, or the Multiple Risk Factor Intervention Trial, cost US$115 million and reported inconclusive results in 1982. This was largely because there was no adequate control group, it being considered unethical to identify people at high risk of developing heart disease and then deliberately fail to give them any advice to help them reduce their risk.

Studies on animals

Animal studies can be a useful way to check out a theory, for example, if scientists think that eating a high-fat diet causes high levels of cholesterol in the blood, they can feed animals very high-fat diets and then measure their blood cholesterol levels. It is also useful to look at the effects of diet over several generations of animals – something we would have to wait centuries to observe in humans. Ultimately, although animal studies add weight to existing evidence, they cannot provide proof of cause and effect in humans.

Laboratory trials

Finally, there are laboratory trials of various sorts, looking at the way that chemicals react together, or at the effect of certain substances or conditions on cells taken from body. This can tell scientists how something might happen inside the body, but there is always the doubt that what happens in a laboratory does not happen in the same way in the body itself.

An impossible solution

The only way to show beyond doubt that one or other aspect of environment played a part in disease would be to run a trial with two groups of people from their birth to their death, with their environments identical in all but one respect. In this way, you could be certain that if one group had a consistently higher rate of a certain disease, this disease must be at least partially caused by the environmental factor in question, because everything else about the groups of people would be identical. Such a trial would be out of the question as not only impractical and unwieldy, but also unethical, since it would mean controlling the participants' entire lives from start to finish. Because of this, experts have to rely on evidence of a less satisfactory sort. Differences of opinion about the degree of certainty this less convincing evidence gives, leads some experts to be more reticent about recommending dietary change than others.

. . . and why they disagree about who should change their diet

The arguments don't stop here; even if the experts were agreed that the evidence indicates some sort of link between diet and health, they would continue to disagree about the scope of the resulting recommendations. Should everyone be encouraged to make appropriate changes to their diet – this is known as the population strategy – or only those who are particularly at risk of developing the disease in question – the high-risk approach?

The fact is that not everyone is likely to benefit from making dietary changes: most of those who are already at high risk of developing the disease are likely to benefit by taking preventive action, and some of those who are at lower risk may benefit, but many people would be taking preventive measures unnecessarily.

Some experts believe that dietary change should not be recommended unless it is known that it will be beneficial to all the individuals in question, by preventing disease and prolonging life. The problem then is to determine which types of people are most likely to benefit from changing what they eat, and then find a way of identifying these individuals in the population, to offer help. Proponents of this approach argue that this high-risk strategy is more cost-effective than the more general population approach, but in fact it could be very expensive indeed to identify all the people who are at high risk from any one disease, particularly if it involved screening the entire population.

Other experts believe that the most effective way to prevent disease is by altering average dietary intakes, by encouraging the entire population to make appropriate changes. Although many of the small number of people at high risk are likely to die of the disease, most of the deaths from the disease will occur in the rest of the population. The disease may not be so common among the lower-risk groups, but since more people are at moderate or low risk than are at high risk, more lives could be saved by influencing the moderate-risk population than by targeting the high-risk group.

For example, two studies of heart disease in the UK found that the fifth of the population at the highest risk of having a heart attack actually accounted for only a third of the heart attacks that occurred. The remaining two thirds of heart attacks were in people at moderate or even low risk. This indicates that the population approach could result in more lives being saved. Moreover, this approach means that over time the habits of the entire population are likely to change, reducing the need for future health education campaigns. But it does mean that many individuals are being encouraged to make dietary changes who may derive no direct benefit.

This may sound like so much semantic detail, but the difference of opinion on high-risk versus population health care campaigns is an important one, because on this issue rests the question of whether each of us would be well advised to take note of what the experts say, or to sit back comfortably and ignore the advice, on the grounds that we are not at high risk of developing any of the diseases in question anyway.

The media view

Although opinion among experts weighs heavily in favour of Britons making changes to their diet, this is not the picture you might get by reading the daily press or even watching television, because the balance of expert views is distorted by the nature of media coverage and the food manufacturers' sponsorship. Journalists are keen to get a news story, manufacturers keen to ensure a continued market for their current products. In an attempt to reassure the public that the food they are selling is healthy, manufacturers provide backing for those scientists who are prepared to say that they don't believe there is enough evidence yet on which to base advice to cut back on sugar or salt, for example.

In recent years, salt and sugar manufacturers have held press conferences featuring scientists who hold views favourable to their products. These conferences have had banner headlines the next day, but they represent only the views of some of the world's experts. The other, less controversial views don't get so much publicity because they don't sell newspapers or foods. Hence most food experts must rely on health education campaigns to spread their views to the public, and relatively little money is available for this sort of promotional activity, compared with manufacturers' promotional budgets.

2
WHAT WE NEED
AND WHAT WE EAT

Food has to provide the nutrients – carbohydrate, protein, fat, vitamins and minerals – required to keep the body in good working order, and the energy needed for activity and growth. But how much of all these do you need?

Recommended Daily Amounts

The Department of Health issues guidelines for the amount of energy, protein and various vitamins and minerals that people should, on average, eat each day. These are the Recommended Daily Amounts or RDAs. The exact amounts of the various nutrients that each individual needs vary according to age, sex, weight, height and physical activity, among other things. RDAs represent goals for the average intake; in other words, if the average intake matches the RDA then the vast majority of the population are eating sufficient quantities of the nutrient in question, although some individuals will be eating a lot more and some a lot less.

RDAs for vitamins and minerals are based on the amount of the nutrient required to protect people from developing deficiency diseases, that is, diseases directly caused by having an insufficient amount of that nutrient. Too little iron, for example, causes anaemia and too little Vitamin C results in scurvy. RDAs are calculated on the basis of an amount required to prevent the related deficiency disease, plus a safety margin. In the case of Vitamin C, an intake of 10 milligrams a day prevents scurvy developing, and that figure has been trebled to give a relatively arbitrary RDA of 30mg.

RDAs for protein and energy are related more closely to average intakes; there are no built-in safety margins. In fact, average protein intakes match the RDA very closely. On the other hand it is generally agreed that energy RDAs are set rather too high (see What we need for energy, below). RDAs are not given for fat or carbohydrate, because, the Department of Health asserts, although they are the major sources of energy, the body needs very little of these from a nutritional point of view.

It is hard to find out how far the British diet matches RDAs and the dietary guidelines suggested by COMA and NACNE; there is no perfect method for measuring what people actually eat. The best guides we have are the National Food Survey and dietary studies of smaller numbers of people. Together these give us a reasonable idea of what people are eating, but there are weaknesses in the data which make it difficult to be absolutely certain how much of certain nutrients people are eating.

The National Food Survey

This is run by the MAFF and involves some seven thousand randomly selected households recording all the food that enters their home during a week. The survey runs throughout the year, so seasonal variations in diet are accounted for. The food records are then analysed for nutritional content.

Although the National Food Survey is a very important source of information about food intakes and especially about trends or changes in patterns of food consumption, it has a number of inadequacies. First, the exercise gives data for whole households, not for individuals. This means we don't know how the diets of different sections of the population vary, for example the old and the young, men and women. The survey doesn't take into account food that is eaten outside the home – school dinners, canteen lunches, business dinners or snacks eaten out of the house, for instance. It includes no allowance for alcohol or soft drinks nor for confectionery bought by individual members of the household and consumed off the premises. All this means that the figures given by the survey are likely to be lower than actual intakes, particularly for sugar, a large amount of which is contained in soft drinks and confectionery.

Dietary studies

These involve a small number of people weighing and describing everything that they eat for between one and seven days. This dietary diary is then analysed for nutritional content.

Studies of this sort are useful for telling us about the diets of particular sections of the population and can also help to confirm the picture given by the National Food Survey, but they also have weaknesses. First, the small number of people about whom they give information may all turn out to have unusual diets. Second, because taking part in a dietary study is so arduous, people often don't record exactly what they eat, or they alter what they eat during the study period, to make life easier, so the data itself may be unrepresentative of the participants' usual diets.

Food tables

Data from dietary studies and the National Food Survey is analysed according to MAFF food tables which give nutritional content for a host of different foods. Thus the surveys are only as reliable as the food tables themselves. The tables (which are being updated as this book goes to press) give very reliable average information about the nutritional contents of fruit and vegetables, meat and standard dairy products, but these sorts of foods can vary enormously in content. For example, potatoes can have as little as 5mg of Vitamin C per 100 grams or as much as 30mg. Also, the categorisation of food can be vague. Whereas the record or diary may indicate a portion of Black Forest gateau, the tables give figures only for gateaux in general. The approximations that are necessary to analyse the records and diaries may be distorting the picture to a small degree.

What we need for energy

The body can obtain energy from carbohydrate, fat, protein and alcohol, but most energy needs are met by carbohydrate and fat, with only 10–13 per cent coming from protein. The current discussions about a healthy diet revolve around exactly what proportion of energy should be derived from each of these sources; NACNE and COMA recommend we should derive only 30–35 per cent of our energy from fat, leave the protein level as it is and increase the amount of energy gained from carbohydrate to fill the gap (see Diagram 1).

Energy is expressed as calories. The measurements are kilocalories (kcal or Calorie) or kilojoules (kJ), 1 kilocalorie being the equivalent of 4.18 kilojoules. A food that is high in energy is therefore high in calories. Yet it is a common assumption that while energy is good for you and the body needs it in large quantities, calories are fattening and so we should eat less.

In a Consumers' Association survey of the general public in 1985, 820 people were asked whether they had heard of a variety of nutrition terms and then whether these aspects of diet should generally be cut back, increased or left at current levels. The confusion about the variety of terms used to describe energy is self-evident (Table 2), and is perhaps hardly surprising, considering that foods are often described as 'high-energy' or 'low-calorie', rather than the less persuasive, but equally accurate 'high-calorie' or 'low-energy'

Table 2: Consumer awareness of food terms

Those who were aware of the term and said . . . (%)	
Calories should be cut down	48
Energy should be increased	50
Kilocalories should be cut down	47
Kilojoules should stay the same	42

Consumer Attitudes to and Understanding of Nutrition Labelling, BMRB, 1985, commissioned by Consumers' Association, MAFF and the National Consumer Council

Diagram 1

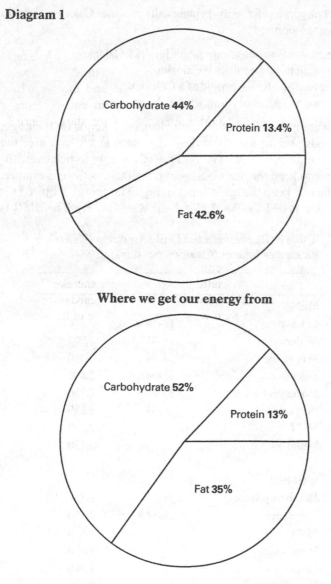

Where we get our energy from

Where we should get our energy from

Household Food Consumption and Expenditure, MAFF, 1986

Carbohydrate, fat and protein all provide Calories, but in different amounts:

- one gram of carbohydrate provides 3.75 Calories
- one gram of fat provides 9 Calories
- one gram of protein provides 4 Calories
- one gram of alcohol provides 7 Calories.

The amount of energy individuals need depends on their age, sex, body weight and lifestyle – the more active you are, the more energy you need. The body needs energy to tick over, for example to keep the heart-beat going, maintain body temperature, breathe and keep the brain functioning. The energy required for all these is called the Basal Metabolic Rate (BMR). The BMR is

Table 3: Recommended Daily Amounts (RDAs) for energy intakes (Calories per day)

	Age	Calories
MEN		
Sedentary	18–34	2,510
Moderately active	18–34	2,900
Very active	18–34	3,350
Sedentary	35–64	2,400
Moderately active	35–64	2,750
Very active	35–64	3,350
65–74		2,400
75 and over		2,150
WOMEN		
Most occupations	18–54	2,150
Very active	18–54	2,500
55–74		1,900
75 and over		1,680
Pregnant		2,400
Breastfeeding		2,750

Manual of Nutrition, MAFF/HMSO, 1985

dependent on body size and the fat to muscle ratio, so for an adult woman the basic daily energy requirement is about 1,300 Calories and for an adult man about 1,600 Calories. Additional energy is needed for growth, for physical activity and during pregnancy and breastfeeding.

It is generally recognised that the RDAs for energy intake (see Table 3) have been set rather too high. Our average intake seems to have dropped as we have become a more sedentary population (see Table 4). Nevertheless, the RDAs serve as a guideline; calorie intakes as estimated from the National Food Survey in 1986 give an average energy intake of 2,070 Calories, as compared with RDAs of between 1,900 Calories for a middle-aged woman and 3,350 Calories for a very active young man.

Table 4: The rise and fall in energy intakes

	(Calories per day)
1950	2,470
1960	2,590
1970	2,600
1975	2,290
1980	2,230
1985	2,016
1986	2,071

National Food Survey, MAFF/HMSO

More or less carbohydrate?

In the 1960s and 1970s there was a preoccupation with slimming, rather than healthy eating. Nutritionists recommended that to lose weight people should count calories, reduce the number of them that they ate and cut back on sugar. The popular re-working of this message was to cut back on carbohydrate, and some specific diet plans even recommended reducing starch. The result is that, whatever the rights and wrongs of the message, most people still think of carbohydrates as fattening and if they want to lose weight, they think of cutting back on bread, potatoes, pasta and rice, and try to eat lean meat and salad in their place.

Changing your diet to lose weight is different from changing your diet for healthy eating purposes, but for most people the two are closely linked. This has made it difficult for us to make the leap from the low-carbohydrate slimming diets of the 1960s to the high-fibre, higher-carbohydrate, overall health diets of the 1980s. It looks to some as if the advice of the 1960s has been completely turned on its head.

The two messages are not in fact contradictory. The confusion can be explained, at least in part, by there being three major types of carbohydrate: sugars, starch and fibre, found mainly in foods from plants – fruit, vegetables, cereals and nuts. The fibre is what gives plants their structure and shape; starch is the plants' stored energy (not unlike our body fat); and sugar is what starch is broken down into, to make the energy available for the plant to use. Nutritionists in the 1960s advised cutting back on sugar; today they advise eating more fibre and starchy carbohydrates in place of high-fat foods.

The role of sugar

Strictly speaking, we don't need to eat sugar – it provides only energy and that is available from other sources. Some sugar is present naturally in foods, for instance fruit and even milk, but what we normally think of as sugar is processed from sugar cane or beet and added to food either at home or, in the case of processed foods, by the manufacturer. Taken as a whole, the various forms of sugar are known as 'sugars'.

Before sugars can be used in the body, they must be broken down into smaller, simple sugars. This process takes place early in the digestive process, starting in the mouth. Once broken down, or digested, sugars travel through the intestine walls and into the bloodstream, which transports them around the body. Cells in the body then break the sugar into carbon dioxide and water, and in so doing energy is released. This process is controlled by hormones, which ensure that a relatively constant level of sugar is available in the blood. Of these hormones, insulin speeds up the transfer of glucose from the blood into cells and glucagon and adrenalin slow it down.

Glucose is the basic type of sugar but there are others: fructose, found in fruit, some vegetables and honey; maltose, which occurs when grains are fermented; lactose, found in milk; and sucrose, which exists naturally and in very large quantities in sugar beet and sugar cane, and in smaller quantities in some fruits and vegetables. Sucrose is a combination of glucose and fructose, and is what we buy as sugar, whether white or brown.

The majority of the sugar we eat is refined or 'added' sugar, added by us, from the packet, or added by food manufacturers to both sweet and savoury foods. It is estimated that, on average we each eat 30–40 kilograms of added sugar per year – that's 80–110 grams or 16–22 teaspoonfuls per person per day.

Total figures for sugar intake are vague. Some estimates are based on the amount of sugar delivered to food retailers and manufacturers in the UK. Other estimates are based on food purchasing habits, as recorded, for example, by the National Food Survey, but, as already mentioned, confectionery and soft drinks, alcohol and foods eaten outside the home are not included in the survey, yet they contribute a very significant amount of sugar to our diet.

A combination of results from dietary studies suggests that sugar provides about 20 per cent of our total energy intake, ranging from about 14 to 26 per cent and including both natural and added sugars. These studies give total sugar intake as between 63 and 141 grams a day, with an average of 104 grams (*Sugars and Syrups Report*, BNF, 1987).

The best estimates for the sources of sugar in our diet give the breakdown shown in Table 5. These figures suggest that 'natural' sugar (sugar that occurs naturally in foods) accounts only for somewhere between 7.5 and, at the most, 30 per cent of all sugar. The remainder is all added sugar, about a third being bought by people as packet sugar and put in tea and coffee, on cereals, or used in cooking, and the other two-thirds added by food manufacturers in processed foods. Thirty years ago these proportions were reversed, with a third coming from processed foods and two-thirds from home cooking and in hot drinks. This represents a big decline in the amount of packet sugar bought, from 25 kilograms per person in 1966 to 11.9 kilograms in 1984, according to the National Food Survey.

Table 5: Sources of sugar in the diet

	%
Packet sugar	35
Preserves etc.	5
Cakes, buns and pastries	3.5
Biscuits	7
Ice-cream	1.5
Soft drinks	8.5
Fresh fruit	5
Canned fruit	1.5
Fruit juice	2.5
Sugar and chocolate confectionery	7
Alcoholic drinks	7
Other	16.5
TOTAL	100.00

Sugars and Syrups Report, BNF, and *National Food Survey*, MAFF, 1984

This seems to indicate that total sugar consumption has fallen; it has, but only by a small amount. In fact, while consumption of packet sugar has decreased, the amounts of sugars (that's all sugars, not just sucrose) used in food manufacturing and processing has increased (see Table 6).

Approximately three-quarters of the sugar added by manufacturers is used to flavour sweet foods – cakes, biscuits, confectionery, desserts, soft drinks and ice-cream, for instance. But about a quarter is added to savoury foods, such as soups and

Table 6: Sugar sales

	Retail sales of packet sugar	Industrial sales	Total sales
1955	1,700,000	1,000,000	2,700,000
1970	1,250,000	1,400,000	2,650,000
1978	1,000,000	1,400,000	2,400,000

The Politics of Food, Geoffrey Cannon, Century Hutchinson, 1987

sauces, to bring out the flavour of other ingredients and to help manufacturers achieve the consistency and texture they think consumers want: 23 per cent of tomato ketchup, for example, is sugar, as is seven per cent of tomato soup, and three per cent of vegetable soup. Even tinned meats, for instance corned beef, have sugar added to make the product softer. Adding sugar can make sauces smooth, cakes lighter and biscuits crumbly. Sugar can also act as a preservative.

The NACNE and COMA reports agreed that we should not eat more sugar than we do at present, and that we should probably eat less. The international consensus is that we should eat about half as much as we do now, and most experts agree that the cuts should be made by eating less added sugar. Foods like fruit and milk, which contain natural sugars, are extremely valuable sources of other nutrients and rather than eating less, we should be eating more of them. Among the added sugars, sucrose in particular is a major culprit in dental decay (see Chapter 7), especially when eaten frequently and between meals.

The overall recommendations on sugar are rather imprecise, but they amount to the following: not to increase sugar intake; to reduce the amount of sugar eaten between meals; and to make any reductions in sugar intake by cutting back on added sugars, not natural ones.

The role of fibre

Called strictly 'dietary fibre', fibre is a combination of several substances that together give plants their shape and structure.

There are two major types: insoluble fibre and soluble fibre. Insoluble dietary fibre includes cellulose, which forms the basis of plant cell walls, and some hemicelluloses, which fill out the plant structure. Soluble fibre includes celluloses, pectins and gums; pectins act rather like cement, holding the plant structure together, whereas gums help plants recover when they are bruised or cut.

All these forms of dietary fibre are forms of carbohydrate, but dietary fibre is also sometimes taken to include a substance called lignin, which is crucial to plant cell structure, providing strength and woodiness. Lignin is totally indigestible and chemically different from all forms of carbohydrate.

Because fibre is composed of so many different substances, it has proved difficult to develop a method of analysing the amount of fibre in food. For food labelling purposes the Government recommends the Englyst method, which gives figures for fibre content that don't include lignin or a substance called resistant starch. However, most food manufacturers label their products according to the Southgate method, which does include these two elements. New MAFF food tables give figures for cereal-based foods using both methods. Until all food manufacturers give Englyst figures, consumers can't reliably compare the fibre content of two similar foods.

Different plants contain the various types of fibre in different proportions. Fruit, for example, contains the most pectin, whereas cereals are high in cellulose. Soluble and insoluble fibre behave in different ways in the body: eating insoluble fibre seems to help prevent constipation and other bowel disorders, whereas eating more soluble fibre might help protect against cancer and heart disease (see Chapter 5). Peas, beans and lentils are rich sources of soluble fibre and cereals are a good source of insoluble fibre, especially wheat, rye and maize.

In itself, fibre isn't a source of nutrition, but foods that are high in fibre tend to contain more vitamins and minerals than their refined equivalents and fibre does help in the process of digestion (see Chapter 5). Because the cellulose walls of plants are particularly high in fibre, eating complete grains, fruits, vegetables and pulses will boost your fibre intake. For example,

100 grams (about 4oz) of apples contains 2 grams of fibre, but the same quantity of apples turned into apple juice contains no fibre at all.

Diagram 2: A grain of wheat

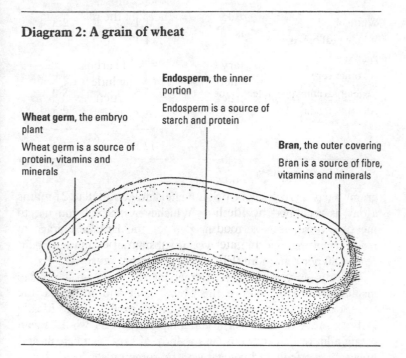

Endosperm, the inner portion

Endosperm is a source of starch and protein

Wheat germ, the embryo plant

Wheat germ is a source of protein, vitamins and minerals

Bran, the outer covering

Bran is a source of fibre, vitamins and minerals

Measuring by the Southgate method, the average British intake of fibre is approximately 20 grams a day (this is the equivalent of about 13 grams as measured by the Englyst method). But people eat very different amounts. When a dietary study carried out by *Which?* in 1985 measured individuals' fibre intakes, it found levels ranging from 6 to 32 grams a day.

Recommendations for the optimum fibre intake are stabs in the dark, based in large part on the average intakes in parts of the world where fibre-related diseases are relatively rare (see Chapter 5). Fibre intakes in countries in the developing world, for example, are between 50 and 120 grams a day. The recommendation for fibre intake in Britain is between 25 and 30

Table 7: Sources of fibre in the average British diet

	By Englyst,	By Southgate,
	grams	*grams*
White bread	1.1	2.8
Wholemeal bread	1.1	1.85
All other bread	0.9	1.95
All other cereal products	2.7	4.0
Vegetables and vegetable products	5.5	8.0
All other foods	1.7	2.8
Total	12.9	21.4

National Food Survey, 1986

grams a day as reckoned by Southgate, and about 18 to 21 grams a day as reckoned by Englyst. Whichever method you use to measure fibre, the increase needed for the British average to reach recommended intake levels is substantial – between about 65 and 80 per cent more than we currently eat.

There is as yet no agreed target for the ratio of soluble to insoluble fibre to achieve the overall goal and maximise the benefit of the two types of fibre. But fibre intake should ideally include some of both sorts and in practice this would mean eating a lot of cereal grains (in the form of breakfast cereals and bread), some fruit and vegetables, and some pulses (peas, beans and lentils).

At the moment the COMA and NACNE fibre recommendations are both single figures for all ages and sizes of people, but it is generally thought that recommendations should vary according to age and maybe calorie intake. The 25–30 gram guideline is probably set too high for old people and is too much to expect children to eat. Both groups have low calorie intakes and eat small weights of food. Eating enough bulk to achieve an intake 25–30 grams of fibre might literally fill up most old people and children so that they would be unable to eat enough other food to gain the other nutrients and calories that they need, in particular protein, vitamins and minerals.

Varying the fibre guidelines according to body weight or calorie intake might give more reasonable goals: for example, 10 grams of fibre for each 1,000 Calories would give goals (by the Southgate method) of 25–30 grams for active adults, 16–21 grams for the elderly, and 10–25 grams a day for children (depending on their age and sex).

Why we need fat, in moderation

Fats are a vital part of the cells that make up our body. Animals and seeds store their reserve energy supplies in the form of fats, just as we do, so fats are first and foremost a source of energy for us. They are made of fatty acids. Some fatty acids can be manufactured in the body but others – known as 'essential fatty acids' – have to be gained from the food we eat because we can't produce them ourselves. So, not all fat is bad.

All fatty acids are made of hydrogen, oxygen and carbon, and the amount of hydrogen they contain affects the way they behave. Fatty acids are either saturated, polyunsaturated or monounsaturated: a saturated fatty acid has as much hydrogen in its structure as there is room for (it is literally saturated with hydrogen); a polyunsaturated fatty acid has four or more spaces that could still be filled with hydrogen; and a monounsaturated fatty acid has just two spaces that could be filled with hydrogen.

All foods containing fat contain some of each type of fatty acid, but they tend to be characterised as being high or low in saturates depending on the proportion of the different fatty acids that they contain. For example, most of the fatty acids in beef dripping are saturated, so it is said to be high in saturates, whereas olive oil is high in monounsaturates, and corn oil and sunflower oil are high in polyunsaturates.

A way to remember the difference is that saturated fats are usually solid at room temperature and polyunsaturates are normally liquid. Also, foods which contain a lot of saturates tend to originate from cows and sheep, for example meats and dairy produce (although hard margarines are also high in saturates, as are many processed foods, like cakes and biscuits). Polyunsaturates tend to be vegetable in origin: nuts and vegetable oils are high in polyunsaturates (except for coconut and palm oils which are high in saturates); there are also some polyunsaturates in wholegrain cereals. Oily fish, such as sardines and mackerel, are particularly high in polyunsaturates.

Some food processing changes the structure of mono- and polyunsaturated fatty acids. This process is called hydrogenation, when the fats are hardened – you may have seen 'hydrogenated vegetable oils' on margarine labels, for example. The NACNE and COMA recommendations are to cut back on total fats, but especially on saturates. However, you might also want to consider cutting back on hydrogenated fats because some experts believe they behave in the same way as saturates.

According to the National Food Survey, average intakes of fat in 1986 were about 98 grams a day, accounting for 42.6 per cent of total average calorie intakes. The bulk of this fat comes in the form of saturated and monounsaturated fats (see Table 8). The majority of the fat we eat comes from dairy foods, meat and meat products and oils and fats (see Table 9).

Table 8: Average daily fat intakes (foods eaten at home)

	grams	% of total calories
Total fat	98	42.6
Saturates	40.6	17.6
Monounsaturates	35.8	15.6
Polyunsaturates	14.3	6.2

National Food Survey, MAFF, 1986

The NACNE and COMA guidance for fat intake is that no more than 30 to 35 per cent of calories should be gained from fat, and that of those calories, no more than 10 to 15 per cent should come from saturated fats. The number of grams of fat that you should eat therefore depends on your calorie intake. Using the RDAs for calorie intake it is possible to work out roughly the maximum amount of fat appropriate for the average person of your age, sex and lifestyle (see Table 10).

Table 9: Where the fat we eat comes from

	%
Oils and fats	28
Meat and meat products	26
Dairy foods	25
Other	14
Cakes, pastries and biscuits	7
Total	100

National Food Survey, MAFF, 1986

Table 10: Recommended fat intakes

	Age	Daily intake
MEN		
Sedentary	18–34	83–98g
Moderately active	18–34	96–113g
Very active	18–34	78–91g
Sedentary	35–64	80–93g
Moderately active	35–64	92–107g
Very active	35–64	116–130g
65–74		80–93g
75 and over		71–84g
WOMEN		
Most occupations	18–54	71–84g
Very active	18–54	83–97g
55–74		63–74g
75 and over		56–65g
Pregnant		80–93g
Breastfeeding		92–107g

One way of expressing the relative amounts of saturated and polyunsaturated fats in the diet is by giving a ratio of grams of polyunsaturates to grams of saturates, called the P/S ratio. In Britain the current P/S ratio is 0.35 grams of polyunsaturates to one gram of saturates, referred to as a ratio of 0.35. It is recommended that this should be increased to 0.45. This would mean reducing the amount of saturates, or increasing the amount of polyunsaturates, or both.

Figures gathered over the last 30 years appear to show that fat intakes have gone down. Daily fat intakes in 1956, for example, averaged 108 grams per person; in 1966, 117 grams per person; in 1986 they were down to 98 grams per person. In fact, although the number of grams has gone down, the proportion of calories gained from fat has gone up – from about 37 per cent in 1950 to 42.6 per cent in 1986 – because overall we are eating fewer calories than before. However, average intakes of the different sorts of fat have been increasing and reducing roughly in line with the recommendations; with saturates going down, polyunsaturates going up and the P/S ratio increasing (see Table 11).

Table 11: Changes in daily fat intake

	Saturates	Polyunsaturates	P/S ratio
	grams	*grams*	
1959	53	9.2	0.17
1969	56.7	11.0	0.19
1975	51.7	10.1	0.19
1980	46.8	11.3	0.24
1985	40.6	13.1	0.32
1986	40.6	14.3	0.35

Diet and Cardiovascular Disease, COMA/DHSS, 1984

The amount of saturated fat that you eat is important because it can have an effect on your blood cholesterol level, and a high blood cholesterol level can in turn increase your risk of heart disease (see Chapter 4).

Cholesterol comes from two sources: it is found in certain foods (for example egg yolks, shellfish and offal), and it can be produced by the liver (80 per cent of the cholesterol in your body is produced this way). The amount of cholesterol you eat is not normally a cause of a high blood cholesterol level, unless you eat an extraordinarily large amount or you suffer from a condition known as familial hypercholesterolaemia. This is because the liver, which is responsible for maintaining blood cholesterol at the appropriate level, is very adaptable; if you eat more cholesterol, the liver produces less, and vice versa.

Cholesterol has emerged as the villain of the fat and heart disease story, but it is worth remembering that a certain amount of cholesterol is essential; for example, cholesterol plays an important part in the production of sex hormones and of bile acids (substances which are present in the bile, which itself aids the digestion of fat).

Protein – not a problem

Eating the right amount of protein is essential to good health but if you are eating sufficient calories for your size and age you will certainly be getting enough protein.

The average protein intake in 1986 (as estimated by the National Food Survey) was 69.3 grams a day or about 13.4 per cent of total energy intake. About two-thirds of this came from animal sources (fish, meat and cheese for example), with the remaining third coming from vegetable sources like pulses, nuts and cereals. In fact, nuts, dried peas and beans contain about the same amount of protein, gram for gram, as meat, fish and cheese, but they account for less of the average intake of protein simply because we tend to eat less of them.

The level of protein recommended by the Government is equivalent to about 10 per cent of total energy requirement, which is an average of about 60 grams a day. The precise figure varies from 54 grams a day for an averagely active woman aged 18 to 54, to 84 grams a day for a very active 18 to 34 year old man.

Protein is made of chains of amino acids, which are the body's building blocks, used primarily for growth and replacement of cells. Any excess protein is turned into energy.

Salt: eating 20 times what we need

Salt is more properly called sodium chloride, of which about 40 per cent is actually sodium. Sodium controls the amount of fluid in the body and since 60 per cent of the body is fluid, sodium plays a crucial role. In turn, the amount of sodium in your body is controlled by the kidneys, which act as a filtering mechanism, cleansing fluid as it travels round the body and through the kidneys. The body also needs sodium for muscle and nerve activity. The action of sodium as a control on the body's fluid content is balanced by the action of potassium, which is found mostly inside the body's cells (sodium is found mostly in the fluids outside the cells, for example in the blood).

Almost all the sodium in the average diet comes from salt, but a small amount is taken in other forms, for instance as the food additive monosodium glutamate (MSG), or as baking soda (sodium bicarbonate). It is estimated that over 95 per cent of sodium eaten is added either at home, in cooking or at the table, or by food manufacturers – very little occurs naturally in foods. By contrast, potassium tends to be found in large amounts in fresh fruit and vegetables, so a diet that is high in sodium may be low in potassium, and vice versa. This has led some experts to suggest that the evidence for an association between high salt intakes and certain diseases could also be taken to be an association between a low potassium intake and the same diseases (see Chapter 6).

Of the 95 per cent of sodium that is added to food, the vast majority (88 per cent) is added by food manufacturers and processors. Salt has been used as a preservative and flavouring for centuries. The Romans called it 'sal' after Salus, the goddess of health, because it had an antiseptic effect, and it was so precious that soldiers were paid in part with a salt allowance –

hence the word 'salary'. Soldiers' rations were cut if they were thought to be 'not worth their salt'.

Since then, food manufacturers have found endless uses for salt. Today salt or a sodium-based additive is added to a host of different foods, for example to cheese, to slow the growth of micro-organisms; to cured meats to preserve, flavour and colour, and to increase the amount of water they will hold; to bread, for flavour, and other baked goods as a raising agent; in solutions of brine for canning vegetables and fish, to preserve and give extra flavour.

Estimates of people's salt intake vary from about 8 to 12 grams, even 15 grams a day. One of the biggest problems with gathering reliable data for salt intakes is knowing how much people add to their own food. The only reliable way to assess salt intake is through dietary studies where the amount of sodium excreted by participants is measured – this gives a very accurate measure of salt intakes, but such studies usually include only a small number of people.

Figures from the National Food Survey show that packet salt is bought at the rate of 2.8 grams (1.11 grams of sodium) per person per day, and 6.7 grams of salt (2.67 grams of sodium) is bought in processed foods per person per day. This gives a total of 9.5 grams of salt and 3.8 grams of sodium a day. But this figure doesn't include foods eaten out of the home and many take-away foods in particular can be quite high in salt. Take for example a hamburger and chips: before you salt the chips, this might contain about 1.8 grams of salt, which could boost daily average intake considerably.

What is clearer than how *much* we eat is where the salt we eat comes from (see Table 12).

Current salt intakes far exceed the body's need for sodium. It is estimated that in a temperate climate such as Britain's, humans require a minimum of 0.5–0.7 grams of salt a day, and in effect we eat around 20 times as much as this. Some experts would argue that our systems have got used to rather more salt than we actually need, and we may even have become dependent on these higher intakes and could react badly to sudden

Table 12: Where the salt we eat comes from

	%
Added at home	12.0
Milk, cream and cheese	9.3
Meat and meat products	18.2
Butter, margarine and other fats	6.9
Vegetables and vegetable products	7.7
Bread	22.2
Other cereal products	11.1
All other food	12.6
Total	100.0

National Food Survey, MAFF, 1986

reductions. But in general, experts consider that it would probably be quite safe to cut salt intakes substantially.

Research on the relationship between salt intakes and disease is not at a sufficiently developed stage to be able to give any clear indication of the optimum intakes of salt (see Chapter 6). But a reduction of 10 per cent, from the current 10 grams a day to 9 grams or so, is generally accepted as being a reasonable starting point.

Vitamins and minerals

The Government produces recommendations for intakes of only selected vitamins and minerals and there is much debate about whether the list should be expanded and whether the levels for those currently listed are set high enough. A Government committee is currently examining these questions. America, for instance, has recommendations for many more vitamins and minerals and sets higher levels.

Table 13: Recommended Daily Amounts for vitamins and minerals

Men	Age	Vitamin A	Thiamin	Riboflavin	Niacin	Vitamin C	Calcium	Iron
MEN								
Sedentary	18–34	0.75 mg	1.0 mg	1.6 mg	18 mg	30 g	500 mg	10 g
Moderately active	18–34	0.75	1.2	1.6	18	30	500	10
Very active	18–34	0.75	1.3	1.6	18	30	500	10
Sedentary	35–64	0.75	1.0	1.6	18	30	500	10
Moderately active	35–64	0.75	1.1	1.6	18	30	500	10
Very active	35–64	0.75	1.3	1.6	18	30	500	10
65–74		0.75	1.0	1.6	18	30	500	10
75 and over		0.75	0.9	1.6	18	30	500	10
WOMEN								
Most occupations	18–54	0.75	0.9	1.3	15	30	500	12
Very active	18–54	0.75	1.0	1.3	15	30	500	12
55–74		0.75	0.8	1.3	15	30	500	10
75 and over		0.75	0.7	1.3	15	30	500	10
Pregnant		0.75	1.0	1.6	18	60	1,200	13
Breastfeeding		1.20	1.1	1.8	21	60	1,200	15

Manual of Nutrition, MAFF/HMSO, 1985

RDAs for vitamins and minerals are related to the level at which deficiency diseases, caused by having an insufficient intake of a certain vitamin or mineral, are rare. In the recent past it has been assumed that vitamin and mineral intakes are no cause for concern in Britain, except for specific groups of people who may be eating relatively small quantities of food and so be in danger of eating too little to gain all the vitamins and minerals they need, for example the elderly and children, or those whose diets are unusual in some respect – notably vegans and some Asians.

There is, however, an increasing concern that low intakes may be quite common, particularly among the poorer sections of society. A dietary study carried out for *Which?* in 1985 analysed the diet diaries of 28 members of the general public and found that there appeared to be cause for further investigation since a high proportion of the group – both men and women – failed to meet recommended intakes of thiamin, folate, Vitamin B6, Vitamin E and zinc. Individual women had rather low intakes of Vitamin A, niacin, pantothenic acid, Vitamin B12 and iron.

Of particular concern was the fact that 11 per cent of the women failed to meet even two-thirds of the RDA levels for thiamin, Vitamin C and calcium; 17 per cent of them failed to meet two-thirds of the recommended levels for riboflavin and niacin; and 28 per cent failed to meet two-thirds of the RDA for iron. Since the sample was very small, this cannot be taken as proof of high numbers of people with vitamin and mineral intake problems, but it is an indication that no one can afford to be complacent about their intake.

The National Food Survey has also shown up a possible iron deficiency, concluding that people in large, low-income families have intakes of only 85 per cent of the RDA for iron. Several other studies have found that people on low incomes are likely to have lower vitamin and mineral intakes in general.

In addition to any problems in achieving current RDAs, some people have suggested that there may be links between the intakes of certain vitamins and minerals and the development of certain diseases and conditions. For example, relatively low intakes of Vitamin A, β-carotene and Vitamin C have all been linked with a high incidence of certain forms of cancer. However, if there is a protective effect, it is evident only at high intake levels – optimum intakes, as opposed to minimum levels. These optimum levels are likely to be much higher than the RDA but it is very difficult to define an appropriate level.

Discussion of vitamin and mineral intakes as a method of disease prevention has not gone as far as discussion about fat, fibre and sugar. And since, in general, a diet that follows current nutrition guidelines would also be higher in vitamins and minerals than the current average diet, higher intakes may be achieved without making specific recommendations.

If, however, dietary advice is misapplied, existing shortfalls in vitamin and mineral levels may be made worse. For example, the 1985 *Which?* dietary study found that when the 28 people tried to change their diets in line with current guidelines and with the help of a nutritionist, they managed coincidentally to increase their intakes of Vitamins B, C and E and iron, but Vitamin A and calcium levels fell among the women. This is probably because in order to cut back on fat, the participants reduced their intakes of high-fat dairy foods, and failed to replace these with low-fat dairy foods, so missing out on calcium, of which dairy foods are a very important source.

3
DISEASES AND DISORDERS

About 70 per cent of deaths in the UK are caused by heart disease, cancer and strokes, which are thought to be at least partly preventable. But some people would argue that reducing the incidence of, say, heart disease, is a wasted effort if the people who would otherwise have died of this, die of something else at a similar age. To be worthwhile, they say, prevention must result in an increase in life expectancy.

Is there a possibility that we could extend our lives by preventing disease, and if so, just how long could we expect to live? In 1900 life expectancy – that is, the number of years that the average person could expect to live – was 45; some lived a lot longer and some died very young. By 1983 life expectancy was 71 for men and 78 for women. This significant increase was achieved because of the long-term effect of major environmental improvements at the turn of the century, for instance improved sanitation, water supplies and housing.

Could life expectancy continue to increase at this rate? Could it be the norm to live to be a hundred in the twenty-first century? The maximum lifespan (that is the longest that anyone has been known to live) is about 115 years. Interestingly, as life expectancy has increased, the maximum lifespan has remained the same – more of us are moving toward the maximum, but it doesn't look as if we are pushing forward the frontier.

Inevitably there will always be some people who die young, either as a result of accidents or incurable disease, and most people are simply physically incapable of achieving the maximum. The maximum average lifespan must take into account all these figures, from a few days' life to 115 years. It is very difficult to say what the average maximum might be, but 85 may be the maximum potential. If this figure is about right, we still have some way to go in extending life expectancy, but not far.

Which diseases could be prevented? Experts in each disease hotly debate the evidence for a connection between environment, and in particular diet, and the evidence certainly varies in strength from one disease to another. In this chapter we give an alphabetical run-down of all the diseases that are thought to be connected with what we eat, no matter how slim the evidence or how few the number of experts who believe in the connection. The evidence is explored in more depth in the following chapters.

Allergies and intolerances

The incidence of food allergy or intolerance is unknown because allergies and intolerances are very difficult to diagnose comprehensively. A recent study carried out for MAFF estimated that at least between 30 and 45 people in 10,000 have an adverse reaction to a food of some sort. Food intolerance is particularly common among young children, especially babies of a few months old, but it seems that well over a third of young children who have a food intolerance stop reacting to the offending foods before they reach the age of two and a half years. In general, food allergy is more likely to occur in people who have other allergic reactions, for example hay fever, asthma or eczema, and in those who have family members who have such allergies.

The term 'allergy' is used to cover a whole range of different conditions that result after contact with a particular substance. Strictly speaking, they should be called 'adverse reactions', and there are several different types of adverse reaction to food; perhaps the easiest differentiation to make is between 'food aversion' and 'food intolerance'.

An aversion is a reaction to a food that occurs only when the person knows what the food is, and is therefore basically an emotional or psychological reaction to a food, perhaps caused by knowing where the food originated. Many people have this sort of reaction to the very idea of eating certain sorts of offal. A food intolerance, in contrast, occurs whether or not the person concerned knows they have eaten the food. Some of the recognised causes of intolerance are:

• an inability to digest certain sorts of food. Some people cannot tolerate lactose, the sugar in cow's milk, for example (this problem is relatively rare in Britain)
• a reaction to certain chemicals, for example caffeine
• a reaction triggered by a substance called histamine that is naturally found in some foods, for example shellfish, strawberries and pawpaw
• an irritant effect on the surface of the digestive system, triggered for example by curry spices or very hot food or drinks
• a true allergy, which means that the body's immune system cannot tell the difference between the food in question and harmful substances from which it would normally defend the body. As a result the immune system attacks the food as if it were a harmful substance and this causes the adverse reaction.

Sometimes people react instantly to the food to which they are intolerant, sometimes they take some time to be affected. The precise nature of the reaction varies considerably, and might include stomach pain, tingling in the mouth or throat, swollen lips, vomiting, diarrhoea, constipation, bloatedness, headache, skin rashes, joint pain, eczema, asthma and sometimes in children, hyperactivity. The most common causes of food intolerance are cow's milk, hen's eggs, fish and shellfish, wheat and other cereals, yeast, chocolate, pork, bacon, coffee and tea.

Why certain people develop intolerances and others never suffer is not at all clear. True allergy tends to run in families, so if one or more of your parents had an allergy of some sort, then you are also more likely to suffer, but whereas they might be allergic to grass pollen or house dust, and suffer sneezing attacks, you might be allergic to aspirin and get skin rashes. Intolerances caused by the inability to digest a certain sort of food or chemical in foods is also likely to be inherited, although just because your mother or father had coeliac disease – an inability to digest gluten in wheat – for example, does not mean that you will also have it.

There is still much debate as to whether frequent exposure to foods known to cause an adverse reaction, especially from a very early age, is likely to cause an intolerance. Some people argue that cow's milk allergy is more likely in babies who have been bottle-fed than in those who are breastfed, and that early weaning on to solids can also be a cause of intolerance, but the evidence is not clear.

Bowel disorders: constipation, irritable bowel syndrome, diverticular disease

Constipation

This is a difficult condition to define, but broadly speaking the faeces are hard and small and defaecation is infrequent. People who are generally constipated have to strain to evacuate their bowels and they may feel that the bowel has not been completely emptied. The incidence of constipation is even more difficult to assess. In one survey of British people, 6 per cent said that they had to strain to defaecate. Another survey of old people showed that 20 per cent complained of constipation and 50 per cent regularly took laxatives. Constipation is undoubtedly eased by increasing the amount of fibre in the diet (see Chapter 5).

Irritable bowel syndrome

This is an equally ill-defined disorder, involving pain in the intestine and alternating diarrhoea and constipation. No one knows how common it is, but a survey of 300 people in Britain showed that 14 per cent claimed to have regular intestinal pain that was relieved by defaecation. Irritable bowel syndrome and constipation account for between 30 and 60 per cent of new cases at gastroenterology clinics. There is some evidence to show that having irritable bowel syndrome makes the development of diverticular disease more likely in the future.

Irritable bowel syndrome seems to be eased with an increase in the amount of fibre in the diet (see Chapter 5).

Diverticular disease

This is rare before the age of 30 and the incidence increases with age; at least one in two people over the age of 80 have it. It is the commonest disorder of the bowel, being present in one in ten people over the age of 40 and in one in three over the age of 60 in the west. The disease is also slightly more common in women than in men.

Diverticular disease has very similar symptoms to irritable bowel syndrome, but is better defined. As waste matter is propelled along, the bowel wall has to sustain substantial pressure. The bowel wall is naturally sturdy to withstand this, but in diverticular disease the wall is weakened and small pouches form in the wall of the intestine, called 'diverticula', making defaecation difficult.

Diverticular disease was rare in Europe during the nineteenth century – it certainly escaped mention in the medical textbooks – but there has been a fairly consistent rise in the number of deaths attributed to it since the 1920s.

Cancer

Nearly one in four deaths in the UK is caused by some form of cancer. Three types of cancer are thought to be particularly likely to be related to diet: bowel, breast and prostate (the gland in men at the back of the bladder). Bowel cancer is the second most common cancer in Britain, accounting for 12 out of every 100 cancer deaths. Among women, breast cancer is the most common, accounting for nine of every 100 cancer deaths. Cancer of the prostate is the third most common cancer among men (after lung and bowel) and accounted for nearly another five of every 100 cancer deaths in 1986 in England and Wales.

In all, there are hundreds of different sorts of cancer, some of which can be treated, for example, skin cancer, and some of which are fatal. Whatever the form, the pattern is the same: the cancer begins with a change in just one cell in the body, and probably in just one of the DNA building blocks that contain the genetic coding of the cell. This tiny change can have a drastic effect on the cell's working; everything that each cell does is dictated by the genetic coding it contains, so if that coding changes in any respect, some aspect of the cell's working will fail or alter.

While the cause of this cellular change is unknown, it may be due to a virus, or the production of a chemical substance of some kind. The cause of the initial cellular change is referred to as an 'initiator'.

The altered cell does not necessarily become a cancer, but can carry on functioning (or malfunctioning) without causing any significant problems. Some altered cells develop into cancers because some substance or circumstance – a 'promotor' – actively promotes the cell's altered development and it begins to reproduce and grow in an uncontrolled way. This results in the cell multiplying at an abnormal rate and the new cells literally mound up, to form a tumour.

The incidence of cancer could be reduced by two routes: either the initiator could be avoided, deactivated or eradicated, or the same could be done for the promotor. A cancer will develop only if both initiator and promotor are present and in this sense both can be said to be causes of cancer.

Different cancers are caused by different initiators and promotors. High fat intakes have been associated with cancer of the bowel, breast and prostate (see Chapter 4). Lack of fibre has been associated with bowel cancer (see Chapter 5).

High intakes of Vitamins C and A and β-carotene have all been linked with low levels of certain sorts of cancer. Vitamin C can inhibit the production of nitrosamines in the stomach, thus reducing the impact of nitrates and nitrites, chemicals used in agriculture and as preservatives in some smoked, pickled and cured foods. In themselves these are harmless, but they can be changed into nitrosamines, which are known to cause cancer in animals. Epidemiological evidence shows a link between a high intake of smoked, cured and pickled foods in Japan and some South American countries and cancer of the stomach, although the evidence goes no further than suggesting there might be some sort of link.

A recent report published by the Food Advisory Committee (which advises MAFF) concluded that the greatest source of nitrites in the UK was drinking water, as a consequence of the seepage of chemical fertilisers into the water supply, from fields used for agriculture. The contribution of food to our intake of nitrites was put at a low level.

Vitamin A helps to regulate the growth of the cells that make up the skin and lining of all the body cavities (epithelial cells). It seems likely that Vitamin A may have some inhibitory effect on the uncontrolled growth that occurs when a cell becomes cancerous – 90 per cent of cancers are epithelial. Some animal experiments have given support to this conjecture.

β-carotene is likely to have a similar effect in relation to cancer as Vitamin A; although we get β-carotene from certain fruits and vegetables, and Vitamin A from liver and certain fats, our system turns any excess β-carotene into a form of Vitamin A which can be stored in the fat in our bodies.

The problem with much of the evidence that links these three vitamins with a lower incidence of certain forms of cancer, is that the studies actually show a link with vegetables that are rich in β-carotene, which are also high in Vitamin C and fibre. This makes it very difficult to know whether the connection is between a low cancer incidence and vegetable intakes, vitamin intakes or fibre, or none of these.

There is an established link between alcohol and cancer of the oesophagus, mouth, throat and larynx. Obesity has also been correlated with the incidence of certain sorts of cancer, especially cancer of the endometrium (lining of the womb). This may be because obesity is also associated with a rise in the hormone oestrogen and high levels of oestrogen can result in cancer of the endometrium.

Doll and Peto (see Chapter 1) estimated that between 10 and 70 per cent of all preventable cancers might be connected with diet in some way. By contrast, tobacco is a factor in the development of about 30 per cent of all cancers, while occupational hazards, pollution, food additives and industrial products are estimated to account for only about eight per cent of all preventable cancers.

Diabetes

Diabetes is a condition in which there is too much sugar in the blood and the body's muscles, which need sugar for energy, are unable to convert it because of a shortage of insulin, a hormone produced by the pancreas. Initial symptoms are extreme thirst, the passing of sugar in the urine, and loss of weight. The disorder affects about one per cent of the UK population and is more common among older people; while about four out of every 1,000 people over the age of 65 have diabetes, only just over one out of every 1,000 people under the age of 22 have the disease. It has become more common in the last 20 years or so, particularly among the young.

There are two types – insulin-dependent diabetes, known as type I, and non-insulin-dependent diabetes, known as type II. Type I is caused by an almost total failure of the pancreas to produce any insulin. No one knows why this happens, but it may be a consequence of something in the immune system. There is no evidence that this type of diabetes is affected by sugar intakes, nor by any other aspect of diet. This type of diabetes tends to occur in people under the age of 30 and accounts for about 25 per cent of all cases of the disorder.

Type II diabetes, the more common of the two types of the disease, is different. Insulin is produced, but not released into the bloodstream in appropriate amounts in response to food. This type tends to run in families and most people who develop it are overweight; obese people are nearly three times as much at risk of developing diabetes as normal weight people. But this does not mean that obesity causes diabetes; both conditions may be a consequence of some other common factor.

A study of identical twins showed that the genetic influence is particularly strong, since when one twin had diabetes, the other almost invariably developed it at a later stage. It seems likely that obesity encourages the development of diabetes in people who already have the genetic tendency to develop it. In one study scientists tried to induce diabetes in prisoners who had no family history of diabetes. They were overfed to make them overweight. Although the 'volunteers' developed higher than usual blood glucose and insulin levels, none actually developed diabetes.

When you eat, your digestive system sets about breaking down the food to release the energy and nutrients that your body needs. The most readily available source of energy is glucose and immediately after a meal the amount of glucose circulating in your blood rises as your system digests food and releases glucose. The level of glucose circulating in your blood is known as the blood glucose level.

The liver can quickly absorb and store much of this glucose as glycogen, but to do so it requires the aid of insulin. As the blood glucose level falls, so the amount of insulin that is produced is decreased. If it falls too low then some of the glycogen stored in the liver is released into the blood stream. In diabetics, for whom the supply of insulin is missing or its action is insufficient, the rise and fall in the blood glucose level as food is eaten is uncontrolled. A substantial rise in the level of sugar in the blood is known as 'hyperglycaemia'.

Gallstones

One study in the UK showed that six per cent of men between the ages of 45 and 59 and 12 per cent of women in the same age group had gallstones – pieces of crystallised bile that can form in the gall bladder. In general, the risk of getting gallstones increases with age, and women have twice the risk of men. Studies looking at the incidence of gallstones in elderly women who had died showed that 30 per cent of them had evidence of gallstones, although this was not generally the cause of their death.

The gall bladder is a small sac attached to the tube that carries bile from the liver into the small intestine. Bile is stored in the gall bladder, ready to help in the digestion of fatty foods.

Gallstones form when the content of the bile is imbalanced, containing too much cholesterol and not enough bile salts, which act as a solvent.

Stones can cause problems if they block either the tube that joins the liver and intestine, or the channel that runs from the gall bladder into this tube. The consequence is a swollen and blocked gall bladder, which can result in jaundice. Gallstones may also cause disease of the gall-bladder wall itself and could lead to cancer of the gall-bladder, although sometimes they are no trouble at all and give no further complications. Studies of people who have developed gallstones show that they are more likely to be overweight and have high blood sugar and fat levels. Equally, people who are overweight or have diabetes are more likely to develop gallstones.

Heart and circulatory disease

Over 48 per cent of deaths in England and Wales in 1986 were caused by some form of circulatory disease, mainly cardio-vascular (heart) disease and cerebrovascular disease (stroke and high blood pressure).

Coronary heart disease (CHD)

This was responsible for nearly 28 per cent of all the deaths in England and Wales in 1986 – that's 163,104 deaths. It is a major cause of premature death in men: 37 per cent of deaths in men between the ages of 30 and 65 are caused by CHD. Not everyone who has CHD is immediately incapacitated, however; a study of over 18,000 British civil servants, which involved screening them to look for signs of CHD, reported in 1974 that the equivalent of 16 per cent of the male population between the ages 40 and 64 had some signs of CHD. This is the equivalent of 1.1 million people.

CHD refers to a range of symptoms collectively caused by harmful changes in the coronary arteries, which supply the heart muscle with blood. In general, the disease results in the arteries becoming narrowed, which means that the blood flow to the heart is impaired.

The precise cause of the disease remains a mystery, but there are a number of factors that are known to make it more likely, principally smoking, high blood pressure and a high blood cholesterol level. Other possible risk factors include diabetes, a family history of CHD, obesity, stress, personality, physical inactivity and even the hardness of tap water.

The heart's function is to pump blood around the body to provide its various parts with oxygen, which is carried in the blood. But the heart muscle itself needs oxygen to function and this blood is transported to the heart in the coronary arteries. In CHD the blood flow to the heart is affected by changes in the artery walls which are the result of a process called atherosclerosis.

The first stage of atherosclerosis occurs when the lining of the artery wall becomes damaged. The body's automatic response is to heal the area, forming a sort of scab for protection. Unfortunately, in atherosclerosis the healing process continues unchecked and as the cells build up in the area, the artery wall becomes thickened and the artery itself becomes narrowed and less elastic – arteries need to be very elastic to withstand the high pressure of blood being pumped out of the heart. This thickened area is known as an 'atheroma' and is made of scar tissue and deposits of fatty materials (lipids) including cholesterol. Atheroma is found in almost all ageing arteries, but atherosclerosis is a consequence of severe narrowing of the arteries.

One result of atherosclerosis is that the heart muscle may be deprived of oxygen and if this happens, one of several things may occur, depending on the duration and extent of the restriction in blood flow: there may be pain or discomfort (angina pectoris); the heart may cease functioning altogether (heart attack); or sudden death may occur.

Angina pectoris causes pain in the chest and sometimes also the neck and left arm. The immediate cause is an increased demand being placed on the heart, perhaps because of exercise or stress. Because the coronary arteries are narrowed, the heart doesn't get the increased blood supply that it needs to cope with the new demands being put on it.

In a heart attack, the blood supply to a part of the heart muscle is stopped altogether for a period of time, and that part of the muscle may die. The extent of the damage to the heart muscle plays a large part in determining whether or not the affected person will survive the heart attack or not. It is generally thought that heart attacks are caused when a blood clot or thrombus forms over an atheroma and blocks the artery, at least temporarily.

Sudden death occurs in people with atherosclerosis that is so severe that it restricts the heart's blood supply. In these cases there may not be a blood clot blocking the artery, nor, in some cases, any previous regular pain.

There is general agreement among experts that changes in lifestyle and environment could reduce the incidence of CHD, but because CHD is a multifactorial disease it is difficult to isolate which changes would be the most appropriate or beneficial. The aspect of diet that is thought most likely to affect the risk of developing CHD is fat intake, in particular saturated fat intake (See Chapter 4). The British rates of death from heart disease are second only to Finland. Over the last 20 years or so most other countries with high rates have managed to make significant inroads into the incidence – the USA, Canada, Australia, New Zealand, Finland and Belgium have all achieved a decline in the incidence of cardiovascular disease by some means or other.

Hypertension (high blood pressure)

At least one in eight of the population has high blood pressure. There is an increased risk of developing the condition if other members of your family have it, although in developed countries almost everyone has increasing blood pressure as they get older. Hypertension is an important cause in at least one third of all CHD and stroke cases.

Blood pressure is literally the pressure that your heart has to apply to pump the blood around your body. Blood pressure changes naturally and necessarily depending on the demands you are making on your body; exercise requires extra supplies of oxygen, which means more blood must be pumped around and so the blood pressure increases. But this increase in blood pressure is not what is known as high blood pressure or hypertension. This occurs when the average resting blood pressure is consistently above normal levels. People who have high blood pressure are more likely to develop CHD and stroke, and high blood pressure also plays a role in the development of kidney disease and certain eye diseases.

Blood pressure is calculated by measuring pressure when the heart is contracting to expel blood (systolic blood pressure) and when the heart is resting between contractions (diastolic blood pressure), and then putting the first figure over the second; a normal reading is 120/80 (mm mercury). In the west there is a gradual increase in blood pressure over age, so that by the age of about 65, normal average blood pressure might be about 160/90 (this increase in pressure with old age is not seen in the developing world). Defining high blood pressure is very difficult, but mild hypertension is generally taken to be when the diastolic pressure is between 90 and 105, moderate hypertension when the diastolic pressure is between 105 and 120 and severe when the diastolic is above 120.

The physical cause of high blood pressure is often that the blood vessel walls are no longer sufficiently elastic to cope with the pressure exerted on them by the heart, or that the blood vessels have become too narrow to take the flow of blood – in other words, atherosclerosis has developed. Since we all develop atherosclerosis over the years, this may explain why blood pressure rises with age. It is also thought that the amount of salt in the diet may play some part in the development of high blood pressure (see Chapter 7).

Cerebrovascular disease

Strictly speaking, this is a disease of the brain and its blood vessels. A little over 12 per cent of deaths are caused by stroke, which is rather more common in women (1,783 female deaths in 1986 compared with 1,134 men). Cerebrovascular disease affects the blood supply to the brain in a similar way to the effect of coronary heart disease (CHD) on the blood supply to the heart. If the blood supply to a part of the brain is temporarily or permanently reduced or cut off, that part of the brain tissue will die. This may result in speech disturbance or paralysis of some part of the body.

Strokes can occur in two ways, either because an artery supplying the brain has become blocked, perhaps by a blood clot, or because the arteries become frail and burst, causing a haemorrhage into the brain tissues. Just as with CHD, atherosclerosis of the arteries supplying the brain makes a blockage more likely. Sometimes blockages are caused by blood clots that have moved around the body, from the heart to the brain, for example. There is a link between CHD and cerebrovascular disease because both are made more likely by atherosclerosis.

Haemorrhages are likely to occur when there are weak spots in the walls of the blood vessels supplying the brain. Some people are born with weaknesses of this sort, called aneurysms, but they are not generally a problem unless the blood pressure increases and puts the weak vessel wall under strain. High blood pressure also has a tendency to produce weak spots in the walls of the very small blood vessels in the brain.

Hiatus hernia

The human trunk is divided into the chest and abdominal cavities by the diaphragm. The only things that run directly from one cavity to the other are the oesophagus (gullet) and the trachea (windpipe). A hiatus hernia occurs when some of the gut slips up into the chest cavity through the hole in the diaphragm via which the windpipe and gullet pass. Often there are no symptoms, but sometimes acid from the stomach will go up the gullet, causing a burning sensation in the throat.

Hiatus hernia is relatively common in the developed world, occurring in 10 to 35 per cent of the population, but in the developing world, only one per cent of the population is affected. It has been suggested that the straining associated with defaecation in constipation, caused by a low-fibre diet, may play a part in the development of this disorder (see Chapter 6). But straining to lift and carry heavy objects might also be expected to have the same effect and the fact that people in the developing world do a great deal of such heavy physical work and yet have a lower incidence of hernia than people in the west, tends to go against this theory.

Overweight

Approximately one in three of the adult population in Britain is overweight to the extent that it is damaging their health. One Government study has estimated that 33 per cent of men and 24 per cent of women are moderately overweight, six per cent of men and eight per cent of women are severely overweight and 0.1 per cent of men and 0.3 per cent of women are grossly overweight (see Chapter 9 for a weight chart and definitions of the grades of overweight). Over the last 40 years or so the average body fat content of the adult population has increased by 10 per cent.

Moderate overweight doesn't carry significant health hazards for people over the age of 50, but in younger people it should be treated. Moderate overweight in the young is associated with increased mortality, there are social disadvantages attached to being overweight and young, and it is anyway easier to treat than more serious degrees of overweight, which might develop if the problem remains untreated.

Energy needs vary substantially from individual to individual, with some people using twice as much energy as others even though they are the same weight and height. This is partly due to differences in levels of physical activity and in body composition – the ratio of fat to lean, for example. There may also be differences between individuals in their response to over-eating which could partly account for the common observation that some people find it much easier to avoid weight gain than others. Recent studies, however, suggest that most overweight people do in fact eat more than normal weight people.

Life insurance tables show that as people's weight increases in relation to their height so their risks of developing a range of disorders increase – heart disease, high blood pressure, arthritis, diabetes, gallstones and even some forms of cancer. If obese people reduce their weight to acceptable levels and manage to maintain it within these limits, they also reduce to normal level their risk of ill health, and they have an average life expectancy. It is widely believed that a high-fibre diet may help people not to gain weight and indeed to lose weight if they are already overweight. It is also suggested that a high-sugar diet is likely to lead people to gain weight (see Chapter 5 and Chapter 8).

Tooth decay

Tooth decay or dental caries occurs when the enamel of milk and permanent teeth is eroded and the soft centre of the tooth which carries the nerves and blood vessels is left open to infection and damage. Tooth decay is predominantly a disease of childhood. In a Government survey carried out in 1983, 48 per cent of five-year-old children in England and Wales had at least some tooth decay, and by the age of 12 an average of 4.3 teeth were affected. The evidence also shows, however, that the incidence is on the decline, by up to 50 per cent, according to some studies in Northern Europe and America.

The plaque that naturally forms on teeth plays a central part in the development of tooth decay. Plaque consists of bacteria in a film of sugars and proteins. It is encouraged to form by the frequent consumption of sugars, by eating soft foods and by poor dental hygiene. Plaque occurs on everyone's teeth, accumulating between meals, during sleep and so on. Once it has formed, the bacteria in it interact with food and drink in the mouth, using some of these substances for their own sustenance. In particular, they appear to use sugar and especially sucrose (see Chapter 7). Sucrose is generally thought to be the substance most likely to encourage dental decay.

When bacteria feed off the sugar, an acid is formed; tooth decay arises when the enamel that covers the teeth is attacked by this acid. The acid softens the enamel by removing minerals from it – de-mineralisation – but decay occurs only if this softening is extensive. Tooth enamel that has begun to soften because of attack from acid, can effectively regenerate itself (re-mineralisation) provided it is free of acid for a reasonable period of time. This is why the frequency of sugar consumption is thought to be an important factor in the development of decay. Tooth enamel can be strengthened against decay or de-mineralisation by adding fluoride to the diet or by painting the tooth surface with fluoride.

Varicose veins

The incidence of varicose veins is somewhat unclear simply because they are an ill-defined condition. But however they are defined, they do appear to be less common in the developing world than they are among people in the west. It has been suggested that they may be caused by a full bowel (in turn caused by constipation) pressing on the veins in the leg and obstructing their flow. Another theory suggests that the straining associated with constipation may increase the pressure in the leg veins and so eventually lead to varicose veins (see Chapter 5).

SECTION II

The evidence in detail

4
TOO MUCH FAT?

Fat is the dietary villain of the twentieth century. The butter and margarine industries have done public battle over it: on the one side the virtues of high-in-polyunsaturate margarine are extolled as women are encouraged to protect their husbands' hearts, while all of us are wooed by the 'welcome back' approaches of the butter industry. What lies behind the advertising hype?

On average, fat accounts for over 40 per cent of our calorie intake. Most of it comes from dairy foods, meat and meat products, and oils and fat spreads, for instance margarine and butter. Most people know about the connection between fats and heart disease, but high fat intakes have also been said to play a role in overweight problems and, perhaps more surprisingly, in the development of cancers of the breast, prostate and colon.

Coronary heart disease

Coronary heart disease (CHD) is a major modern killer; it accounts for over one in four deaths in the UK and is the commonest single cause of death. In general terms, having CHD means that your arteries have narrowed and the blood supply to your heart muscle is impaired. The result could be chest pain (angina) when you exercise, or a heart attack as a result of damage to the heart muscle, because it is short of blood; between a quarter and a third of heart attacks are fatal. CHD cannot be cured, although the symptoms can be alleviated and the progress of the disease can be controlled.

Eating too much fat, especially saturated fat, encourages narrowing of the arteries supplying the heart and coronary heart disease may develop. But does that mean that keeping saturated fat levels low will prevent coronary heart disease from developing? Most experts think there is a good chance that it will, but a small number disagree. What they all agree on is that: a high blood cholesterol level is linked to increased risk of coronary heart disease; blood cholesterol levels can be reduced by cutting down on the saturated fats in the diet; and reducing blood cholesterol levels in men who already have a high blood cholesterol level, reduces their risk of developing CHD.

Taken as a whole, the evidence for a connection between saturated fat intakes and the risk of heart disease is strong, but the outstanding question is whether keeping cholesterol levels low will prevent heart disease occurring.

High blood cholesterol levels are linked with CHD

In countries where the blood cholesterol levels are generally higher than elsewhere, the heart attack rate is also higher, and in countries with a generally low level of blood cholesterol, the rate of heart attack is much lower (see Diagram 3). Comparisons of blood cholesterol levels and heart attack incidence have been repeated for a variety of countries and the same picture always emerges. The World Health Organisation went so far as to say in their 1982 report, *Prevention of Coronary Heart Disease*, that, 'The Expert Committee knew of no population in which CHD is common that does not also have a relatively high mean level of total cholesterol.'

The most famous study was the Seven Countries Study in which Ancel Keys compared data from the USA, Finland (both with a high incidence of CHD), Yugoslavia, Japan and Greece (with low levels of CHD), and Italy and Holland. He compared lifestyles and the incidence of CHD in all these countries and found a link with blood cholesterol and consumption of saturated fats.

Variation between countries can sometimes be explained by genetic differences between communities. But people who move from countries with a low average blood cholesterol and low rates of CHD (such as Japan) to countries with high average blood cholesterol levels and high rates of CHD (especially the USA) have an increase in blood cholesterol and heart disease as they gradually adopt the lifestyles and habits of their host country, illustrating that CHD is at least partially a result of environmental influences.

Diagram 3: Blood cholesterol and coronary heart disease

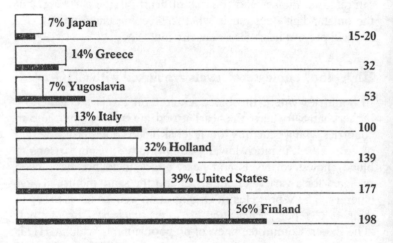

7% Japan — 15-20

14% Greece — 32

7% Yugoslavia — 53

13% Italy — 100

32% Holland — 139

39% United States — 177

56% Finland — 198

☐ Percentage of men with blood cholesterol above 250mg/100ml

■ Average number of men per 10,000 in study who developed CHD during each year of trial

Coronary Heart Disease in Seven Countries (study of men aged 40–59), 1970

The higher the blood cholesterol, the greater the risk of CHD
In general terms, people with a high blood cholesterol level are more likely to have a heart attack than people with low blood cholesterol levels. In fact, the higher the blood cholesterol level,

the more magnified the risk and vice versa. For example, in one American study, twice the blood cholesterol level indicated a fivefold increase in the risk of heart attack. A study in Britain showed that men with blood cholesterol levels in the highest fifth of the population were more than three times more likely to develop CHD as men with blood cholesterol levels in the bottom fifth.

That very high blood cholesterol levels lead to very much increased risks of heart attack is also confirmed by evidence from the one in 500 people who have the rare inherited condition called familial hypercholesterolaemia. These people lack the normal mechanisms for maintaining a fairly constant blood cholesterol level, have blood cholesterol levels of two to three times the average population and are eight to ten times as much at risk of suffering a heart attack.

Will you develop heart disease?

It might seem that measuring blood cholesterol levels would allow a doctor to forecast your risk of developing CHD, but unfortunately the matter isn't as simple as that. If you have a high blood cholesterol level it doesn't necessarily mean that you will develop heart disease. Two-thirds of men with high blood cholesterol levels do not get CHD within 20 years. Some people who have low or moderate blood cholesterol levels may still have a heart attack, while others have high blood cholesterol and have no symptoms of heart disease at all.

The most commonly accepted explanation for this is that genetic differences play some part in an individual's risk of developing heart disease. Someone with a genetic tendency to develop CHD but only a moderate blood cholesterol level may be more likely to develop CHD than someone with no genetic tendency but a much higher blood cholesterol level.

Not all cholesterol is bad

There is more than one type of blood cholesterol and it seems that while one sort is linked with a high incidence of CHD, a second type might actually help to reduce the risk. Cholesterol is transported in the blood by a combination of lipids (fats) and proteins called lipoproteins. Most cholesterol is transported in what are called low-density lipoproteins (LDLs) and a high level of LDLs is a risk factor for CHD. But a small amount of cholesterol is carried in high-density lipoproteins (HDLs) and these do not seem to play a role in the development of CHD. HDLs may in fact serve a protective purpose – the more of them there are, the lower the risk of CHD.

Recent research has suggested that although a diet high in polyunsaturates and low in saturates reduces blood cholesterol levels, the intake of monounsaturates is also important. High intakes of polyunsaturates may reduce the levels of beneficial HDLs, while high intakes of monounsaturates appear to reduce levels of LDLs and maintain or increase HDLs.

In general, then, blood cholesterol levels and heart attack seem to be linked in some way. But in the absence of proof that high blood cholesterol levels cause CHD, it is just possible that the link is a coincidence. Perhaps a third factor is causing both the raised blood cholesterol levels and the increased risk of heart disease.

Clearly blood cholesterol levels are influenced by some environmental factor, otherwise they would not vary so much from country to country or alter when people migrate. There is good reason to suppose that cholesterol levels are affected by the amount of fat in the diet, especially the amount of saturated fat.

The Seven Countries Study showed that the higher the saturated fat intakes, the higher the average blood cholesterol levels (see Diagram 4). In fact, controlling saturated fat intakes can affect blood cholesterol levels; in a 12-year study among patients in a mental hospital in Finland, a diet that was low in saturated fat and cholesterol and high in polyunsaturates resulted in a decrease in blood cholesterol levels. It is generally agreed that a diet that is high in saturated fats increases blood cholesterol levels and one that is high in polyunsaturates decreases blood cholesterol levels.

Diagram 4: Blood cholesterol and saturated fatty acids

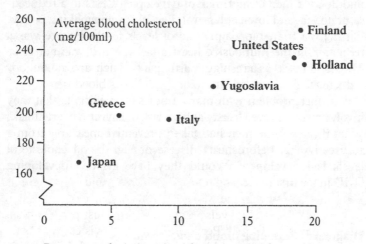

Percentage of calories gained from saturated fatty acids

Coronary Heart Disease in Seven Countries (Study of men aged 40–59), 1970

Reducing high blood cholesterol levels reduces the risk of CHD

If people who already have a high blood cholesterol level take action to reduce it, they reduce their risk of developing CHD and suffering a heart attack (see Diagram 5). Unfortunately, most of the trials that have shown this suffer from a fundamental weakness: the participants have been encouraged not just to cut back on saturated fat, but also to use cholesterol-lowering drugs where appropriate. Trials of this sort concentrate on people who are already at very high risk of heart attack because they have particularly high blood cholesterol levels and, not wanting to put these people at any additional risk, the organisers quite reasonably try every possible method of reducing the risk of CHD. The Oslo Trial, for instance, introduced over 1,200 middle-aged men at high risk of developing CHD to a reduced-saturated-fat and low-cholesterol diet, plus a no-smoking policy. During the trial, blood cholesterol levels fell and there was a reduction in the number of heart attacks, but it was not clear whether this was as a result of participants giving up smoking, or reducing their saturated fat intake.

A further problem with many studies of this sort is that they involve men who are already at high risk of having a heart attack. What if these same men had taken preventive measures from a very early age, before heart disease or high blood cholesterol levels had developed? Would they have avoided developing CHD in the first place?

Diagram 5: Reducing blood cholesterol

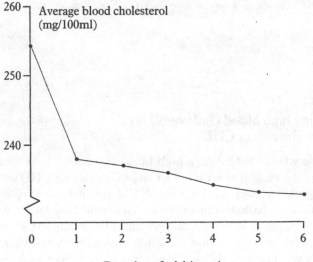

Duration of trial (years)

Multiple Risk Factor Intervention Trial, JAMA, 1982

The only way to assess the effect of reducing saturated fat intakes as a preventive measure is to monitor a group of ordinary people over an extended period of time. All the trials of this sort have been inconclusive. Community prevention trials, where the entire population or a specific group of people is asked to change their diet regardless of their risk of developing CHD, have shown that it is possible to reduce the risk factors for CHD through health education. For example, the North Karelia Study (see Chapter 1) set out to reduce the incidence of smoking and lower blood cholesterol levels and blood pressure by a process of public education with back-up services, such as no-smoking support groups and the promotion of certain sorts of foods in shops. CHD incidence fell, but unfortunately, because of a fault in the trial design, it wasn't possible to tell whether the health education effort was responsible.

A World Health Organisation Collaborative Trial showed that reducing risk factors for CHD could reduce the incidence of the disease, but this trial employed dietary change, no-smoking policies, weight reduction, exercise and treatment for blood pressure, and the results were mixed. The trial involved 60,000 people in 80 factories in Belgium, Italy, Poland and the UK. The people in half the factories were given advice and, where appropriate, treatment; the others acted as controls. Overall, there was a reduction in the incidence of CHD, but the figures varied from one country to another. In Britain there was only a very small reduction in risk factors, and so, not surprisingly, no reduction in CHD incidence.

Many of the weaknesses and inconsistencies of trials like these can be explained, but there is nevertheless room for a small number of people to claim 'case not proven'. True, there is no evidence which proves conclusively that reducing saturated fat intakes will reduce the incidence of CHD. But will there ever be such conclusive proof? Of all the cases for a relationship between diet and disease, the evidence for saturated fat intakes affecting the risks of CHD is second only to that for sugar and tooth decay. The few dissenting voices have had a disproportionate amount of media attention.

Cancer

Nearly one in four deaths in the UK is caused by cancer and the cancers that have been associated with the amount of fat we eat – cancers of the breast, prostate and bowel – are some of the most common. Breast cancer is the most common cancer among women, prostatic cancer is the third most common cancer in men and bowel cancer is the second most common cancer overall, second only to lung cancer in men.

Breast cancer

Several international comparisons have shown a strong association between fat intakes and breast cancer incidence (see Diagram 6). But if fat intakes affect the risk of developing breast cancer, it is fat intakes in childhood and adolescence that appear to have the greatest impact. Women who migrate from countries with a low fat and low breast cancer incidence, for instance Japan, to countries with a high level of both, for instance the USA, become more at risk from breast cancer as they adopt the lifestyle of their host country, but it is only when one or two generations of Japanese women have lived an American lifestyle from birth that the increased incidence of breast cancer is fully developed. Japanese immigrant women initially don't have the same incidence of breast cancer as their American counterparts.

One weakness in all the studies of fat intake and breast cancer is that since fat is high in calories, increasing the amount of fat in the diet tends also to increase the calorie content. This means that the association between fat and breast cancer might actually prove to be one between a high calorie intake and breast cancer. There is certainly a higher incidence of breast cancer in obese animals, and restricting their calorie intake inhibits the development of the cancers. Of course, cutting back fats is one fairly easy way to reduce calories.

Diagram 6: Fat consumption and breast cancer

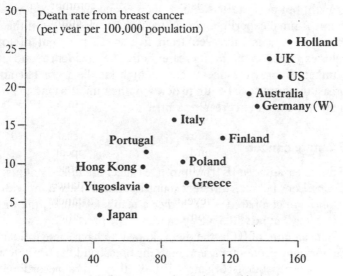

The Causes of Cancer, OUP/Journal of the National Cancer Institute, Vol 66 June 1981 © Doll and Peto, 1981

Are you at risk?

Having a high fat intake doesn't necessarily mean that you will develop breast cancer, but it makes it more likely. Comparisons of individuals' fat intakes and breast cancer incidence have not shown a clear link between the two. This may be because the studies have relied on information about fat intakes at the time of the study, whereas fat intakes earlier in life might be more significant. It could also be that, as with CHD, there is some genetic complication. Some people may simply be more likely to develop breast cancer, whatever they do. ‚

It may also be that a high-fat diet promotes breast cancer – some other initial cause may be required to set off the cancer growth, but once started, a high-fat diet encourages its development. Animal experiments tend to support this theory: if the fat intake of rats is increased from five to 20 per cent of total calories, this tends to increase both the incidence and the number of breast cancers, and if high-fat diets are fed after breast tumours have begun to develop, the tumours tend to grow more quickly and in greater number.

Prostate cancer

Fat intakes and deaths from prostate cancer are linked not just in comparisons between different countries, but also when individual intakes are compared – the higher a man's fat intake, the more likely it is that he will develop cancer of the prostate.

The amount of fat in the diet is known to have some influence on hormone production, and both the breast and the prostate are hormone-dependent organs (that is, they work according to instructions issued by hormones). It may be that an explanation of the effects of fat on these cancers could be found by looking at hormone production.

Bowel cancer

There seems little doubt that cancer of the bowel is related in some way to one or more aspects of diet, but the problem is in determining which aspects of diet are most relevant. Connections have been made between bowel cancer and fat, saturated fat, high calorie intakes, and low fibre levels. The evidence of a link with fat is certainly less conclusive than that for a link with fibre, but since low-fibre diets tend also to be high-fat diets, it could be that the condition is related to both these.

There is more information about bowel cancer in Chapter 5, but here we give a brief run-down of the evidence for a link with fat intakes.

Comparisons between countries show links between the incidence of bowel cancer and deaths caused by it, and fat intakes. But there is no clear link between an individual's intake and the risks of developing the disease: studies give conflicting and unclear results. This may be because the variation in average fat intakes between countries is much greater than the variation between individuals' intakes within a single country. Also, many of the studies quoted by experts were not designed to assess possible links between fat and bowel cancer. Not surprisingly, the strongest links have been shown in studies that *were* designed specifically for this purpose.

Evidence gathered about the normal diets of people who have already developed bowel cancer is equally confused. Several studies have found that patients had a higher consumption of high-fat foods, but other studies point to a link with saturated fats and yet others implicate not just total fat intakes but also low fibre intakes.

It could be that, as with breast cancer, cancer of the bowel is initiated by some non-dietary factor, but diet then encourages the cancer to develop. When bowel cancers are encouraged to develop in laboratory rats, the incidence and number of cancers increases as the amount of fat in the diet is increased. However, since high-fat diets also tend to be low in fibre and high in calories, it may be that this evidence for connections between fat intakes and cancers of the bowel may actually be evidence for a relationship between fibre intakes or high calorie intakes.

From a physiological point of view, it seems perfectly reasonable to suggest that fat plays a role in bowel cancer, since fat affects the nature of the food residues that pass through the bowel. The more fat in the diet, the more bile acids and steroids the liver produces to help digest the fat. People in countries with either a high or a low risk of developing bowel cancer tend to have a higher concentration of bile acids in body waste. It could be that chemicals in these bile secretions play a part in the development of bowel cancer.

In general, then, the bowel cancer/fat theory seems to make sense, but there is a long way to go before it is widely accepted.

Overweight

Obesity, or being overweight, is a consequence of excess consumption of calories and is not caused by a high-fat diet alone. But fat contains more calories gram for gram than carbohydrate or protein and so it is easy to eat more calories in the form of foods that are high in fat than it is calories in the form of high-fibre carbohydrate foods. For example, 200 Calories'-worth of Cheddar cheese weighs 49 grams (1.7 ounces), while 200 Calories'-worth of wholemeal bread weighs 93 grams (3.25 ounces) – a lot more to eat. Cutting back on fat should make it easier to lose weight and maintain the reduction, partly because of the calories you are avoiding and also because you will need to replace some of the calories gained from fat with carbohydrate foods, preferably high-fibre ones, which have their own weight-loss advantages (see Chapter 5).

5
NOT ENOUGH FIBRE?

Fibre is the substance that gives plants their shape and structure – the equivalent of flesh and bones. In the past humans have eaten a lot of fibre and average intakes in the developing world range from 50 to 120 grams a day, but in the west today we eat relatively little (an average of 20 grams a day in the UK). The modern western diet contains a great deal of processed food from which the fibre has been removed: white bread, corn flakes and white rice, for example. To boost fibre intakes we would need to eat more of the less processed foods, such as wholemeal bread, brown rice and wholegrain-type cereals.

Increased public awareness of fibre can probably be dated from the publication in 1982 of Audrey Eyton's book, *The F-Plan Diet* (Penguin Books), which advocated a high-fibre diet as the healthiest and easiest method of losing weight. It used as its evidence a 'popular' version of a report published in 1980 by the Royal College of Physicians, called *Medical Aspects of Dietary Fibre*. But the advantages of a high-fibre diet aren't limited to controlling overweight; according to many experts, fibre also has a role to play in the treatment of a range of different conditions, including: diabetes; constipation; a variety of bowel and intestinal complaints affecting excretion; bowel cancer; dental disease, and even coronary heart disease.

Discussion about the benefits of fibre in the diet is not new: in the fifth century BC, Hippocrates (after whom the Hippocratic oath, to which doctors still adhere, was named) wrote, 'Wholemeal bread cleans out the gut and passes through as excrement.' The case for fibre has gained momentum since the 1950s, when a number of scientists suggested that dietary fibre might protect against far more diseases or conditions than simply constipation.

Interestingly, all three of the key scientists in this debate, Burkitt, Trowell and Walker, had spent a lot of time working in the developing world, where the normal diet is very high in fibre (even if it is also too often deficient in calories) and where the most common causes of death are quite different to those in the west.

Fibre, it has been claimed, has a considerable effect on the way in which food passes through our body. According to some experts, fibre:

- alters the length of time it takes for food to pass through us
- alters the type and number of bacteria that are naturally present in the bowel (rectum and colon)
- can modify the way that fats, sugars, and some minerals and vitamins are absorbed
- can influence the appetite
- absorbs toxins.

What is the evidence for all these different effects and how do they affect our chances of developing diseases?

Overweight

In the west, one in three people is overweight. And this doesn't mean feeling uncomfortable in a pair of tight jeans, this is serious overweight that may have an effect on your health – increasing your risks of suffering from heart disease, high blood pressure, arthritis, diabetes, gallstones and even some forms of cancer.

It is claimed that pursuing a high-fibre diet is the easiest way to lose weight and the best way to maintain weight loss. The truth, or otherwise, of this claim rests on an answer to the question of whether the amount of energy that people consume is affected by the types of foods that they eat. In particular, does eating a high-fibre diet mean that you eat less?

Fibre-rich food is eaten more slowly, satiates the appetite more quickly, leaves you feeling full for longer and gives you a lower blood sugar level (see below). This suggests that the texture of high-fibre foods limits the amount that you can comfortably eat. But this commonsensical assumption has proved difficult to show in experiments, partly because you can't feed people a high-fibre diet without them being aware of it; when subjects of a study know how their diet is being changed it is likely to invalidate the results.

Longer to eat

Fibre-rich foods require more chewing than their fibre-depleted equivalents. This is because food is not swallowed comfortably unless it is soft and moist and high-fibre foods need a lot of chewing to render them soft and moist. Eating a meal's worth of calories in the form of wholemeal bread, for instance, takes 45 minutes, whereas to eat the same number of calories in the form of white bread takes only 34 minutes. In one experiment, half a set quantity of apples was prepared as apple juice and half as purée. The juice was consumed 11 times faster than the same quantity of apples eaten in their raw state, and four times faster than the purée. The amount of chewing that's needed and the length of time it takes to eat high-fibre foods may have an effect on the amount that people eat.

More filling

The amount of effort that is involved in eating has more than a physical significance, it also has a psychological effect – if it is harder work to eat a food, less of it tends to be eaten. For example, when a group of students were asked to drink milk shakes through straws with different sized holes, those with the wider straws drank more milk shake.

Chewing also slows down the rate at which people eat, which may also reduce the amount that they eat. For example in one experiment, obese people were asked to take smaller mouthfuls and deliberately chew very thoroughly. The result was that they ate less, without being conscious of doing so.

People's subjective assessment of their own feeling of fullness also varies, depending on the form in which they eat food. In the apple experiment, the whole apples were considered to be much more filling that the apple purée or juice, and the purée was considered to be more filling than the juice – although all three contained the same number of calories. If high-fibre foods are more filling, they may affect the amount that we eat.

Greater volume

The volume of food in the stomach is greater with foods that contain a lot of fibre, because fibre swells in water. The amount of water that fibre can hold depends on the type of fibre; pectin, for example, holds more water than some other types, and coarsely ground fibre holds more water than more finely milled versions. Quite apart from any fluid that you may drink with your food, there is likely to be more fluid available when you eat fibre because the more you chew food, the more saliva you produce and this extra fluid is swallowed, adding to the food's bulk. The volume of food in the stomach is further increased by extra secretions from the stomach, and the starch in high-fibre foods.

The increased volume of high-fibre foods may have an effect on the amount that people eat and the speed at which waste matter passes through the body (see Constipation, below).

But does following a high-fibre diet mean you actually eat less food? The answer is that this is likely, but it is proving very difficult to show conclusively. The problem is that studies which have looked at the effect of high-fibre diets on weight loss have generally found some other potential cause for any energy reductions that have occurred – a reduction in fat or sugar intakes, or an increase in exercise, for example.

During the Second World War a national flour was introduced as a part of the rationing system, replacing the previously more common white flour. Fibre intakes doubled, energy intakes fell and weight did tend to become lower. But this was perhaps hardly surprising, as people were generally eating less and working harder, often doing more physical work than previously.

When people have been given bran supplements to increase their fibre intake they have rarely produced consistent weight loss. And where there has been some weight loss, it could be explained by a reduction in energy caused by a lowering of fat and sugar intakes.

If eating a high-fibre diet affects energy intakes, it seems most likely that this is because high-fibre foods tend to be more bulky and so it is difficult to eat so much of them. Overweight people asked to follow a high-fibre diet found that their average energy intake fell by 22 per cent without them being aware of eating any less. They had been told that they could eat as much of anything they liked except that for the first seven weeks they were given a ration of fruit and vegetables and wholegrain cereals (all high-fibre foods), while in the second period of seven weeks they were banned from eating any refined carbohydrate foods like white bread, and could eat unlimited amounts of high-fibre equivalents, like wholemeal bread.

Fewer calories available

Another way that eating fibre may affect energy intakes is if the fibre stops the body from using some of the calories in food. The body does not in any case use all the calories that are in food; some food energy goes straight through. But is this amount affected by the quantity of fibre in the diet?

The answer seems to be yes, but in a normal diet the reduction is so small as to make little real difference. In one study, people were given a diet in which 74 per cent of the calories were gained from wholemeal bread. This most unusual, but very high-fibre diet resulted in a reduction of 8.3 per cent in the amount of energy that was made available for the body to use. On the other hand, when people increase fibre intakes by rather more realistic figures of around 10 grams or so, the amount of energy that is excreted rises only very slightly, and most of this lost energy is made up for by eating rather more food in the first place.

There is, then, nothing about a high-fibre diet that will inevitably result in weight maintenance, let alone weight loss. Following a high-fibre diet does not mean you will necessarily eat fewer calories, nor will you excrete sufficient extra calories to make much difference to the number absorbed by the body.

However, it does seem that eating more high-fibre foods is likely to make it easier to reduce or control your calorie intake, simply because high-fibre foods need to be chewed rather more than their refined equivalents and because they hold water and so leave you feeling fuller for longer.

Constipation and other bowel disorders

Constipation, irritable bowel syndrome and diverticular disease are all disorders affecting excretion and it is clear that a high-fibre diet will usually help to ease the symptoms of all three, because fibre increases the bulk and speed of excretion and so makes it easier and more regular. The question, though, is whether a low-fibre diet is the cause of any or all of these conditions.

Greater bulk

The volume of waste matter excreted from the body is increased with a high-fibre diet. In the UK the average weight of faeces excreted each day is about 100 –150 grams. British vegetarians, who tend to have a higher-fibre diet, excrete an average of 225 grams a day, but the average daily weight of faeces in Northern India, Uganda and Kenya (where the normal diet is very high in fibre) is between 311 grams and 520 grams. The amount of extra bulk depends on the type of fibre that is present; in general, cereal fibre adds more bulk than fruit and vegetable fibre.

Faster passage

More bulk also means that the waste passes through the bowel more quickly. For example, studies on groups of Africans showed a transit time of between 36 and 40 hours, whereas in Britain the average transit time is between 40 and 100 hours. A study of British schoolboys gave a transit time of an average 70 hours, whereas in rural African schoolchildren the average was 33 hours. Waste matter is propelled through the intestine by rhythmic contractions in the muscular wall of the intestine and the bulkier the waste matter, the easier it is for the intestine to push it through the system.

It generally takes food about six hours to travel through the stomach and small intestine to the bowel or large intestine. The remainder of the time that waste matter is in the body is spent in the bowel. Here certain remaining nutrients and especially water are extracted, with the result that the longer the waste is in the bowel the less water it contains, the smaller its bulk and the more difficult it is to propel through the bowel.

Irritable bowel syndrome

Fibre seems to standardise the rate at which waste passes through the system and since one symptom of irritable bowel syndrome is alternating diarrhoea (too speedy a passage) and constipation (too slow a passage), it seems reasonable to assume that fibre depletion plays some part in its development. In different individuals, a high-fibre diet increased transit time from one day to two days, and reduced it from three to two days.

Whatever the cause of irritable bowel syndrome, it is clear that increasing the fibre content of the diet of sufferers helps and most doctors now treat their patients with a change in diet.

Constipation

Since there is no reliable method for measuring the incidence of constipation (see Chapter 3) it is almost impossible to compare its incidence in different countries. All experts can cite is the fact that faeces of people in rural Africa and India are bulkier and softer than those of the average Briton.

In general, increasing the amount of fibre in the diet usually relieves the symptoms of constipation, and studies of old people, in particular, show that increasing the fibre content of the diet means that laxatives that may have been taken for some years, can be abandoned.

Piles (haemorrhoids), varicose veins and hiatus hernias may

be linked to needing to strain when passing a stool. If this is the case then a diet high in fibre (which results in a bulkier and softer stool which is easier to evacuate) may also reduce the incidence of these conditions.

Diverticular disease

The incidence of this disease varies considerably, being generally more common in the west and in urban areas than in the developing world and especially in rural areas. Although there seems to be a link with fibre intake, it seems that something more than fibre is the cause. Non-vegetarians with diverticular disease eat less fibre than do vegetarians suffering from it – so far so good – but non-vegetarians without the disease, also eat less fibre than vegetarians who do have the condition. All this suggests that if there is a link with fibre it is not a straightforward one. Nonetheless, studies with rats and rabbits have shown that feeding a low-fibre diet can induce the development of diverticula.

As with irritable bowel syndrome, a high-fibre diet helps people with diverticulitis and most doctors would now recommend it for their patients.

Diabetes mellitus

Diabetes affects one in a hundred of the population, but it tends to affect the elderly in particular; four out of each hundred people over 65 have diabetes. It seems that people are born with a tendency to develop diabetes, although being overweight can then encourage the condition to develop. In diabetics the normal mechanisms for controlling and regulating the amount of sugar that is in the blood, do not function properly. The question is whether what you eat, and in particular the amount of fibre you eat, has any effect on the control of blood sugar levels. The answer is that it does if you already have diabetes, but it is less likely to be a direct cause of diabetes.

Slower digestion

In general, foods that are in a liquid form are digested quickly and travel through the stomach speedily, while the more solid a food, the slower its digestion and passage. This means that the nutrients bound up in a solid food will be released more slowly into the blood. So, for example, half an hour after eating a relatively high-fibre food like wheat flakes, the level of glucose in the blood is lower than after eating the equivalent amount of a more refined, smaller-particle food like white bread. The bread is digested more quickly and the glucose it contains is released in a short space of time, whereas the wheat flakes are digested slowly and the glucose they contain is released over a longer period of time. Soluble fibre, and especially fibre from oats and pulses, has the greatest effect on blood sugar levels.

Fibre doesn't just affect the rate at which sugar is released from food into the blood, but also the rate at which it is cleared away. The amount of sugar that is circulating in the blood is controlled by a hormone called insulin (see the Diabetes section of Chapter 3), and the amount of fibre in food may have an influence on the amount of insulin that is produced. In the apple study (see page 81) the apples, apple purée and apple juice all resulted in a similar rise in blood sugar level. But when people ate apples, the blood glucose level gradually dropped back to its previous level, while in those drinking apple juice, blood glucose levels fell below this previous level.

This excess reduction in blood sugar level is known as rebound hypoglycaemia. In this study the hypoglycaemia remained for three hours with a higher level of insulin than would be normal. This suggests that the less fibre there is in a food, the more insulin is produced in response to it, with the result that the blood sugar control mechanism can be rather too efficient, clearing away too much sugar and leaving the blood low in sugar.

In addition, rebound hypoglycaemia may have some influence on appetite (since blood sugar levels play a part in signalling hunger) and this may be another way that fibre has a role to play in the development and/or control of overweight.

Fibre is particularly likely to help control Type II diabetes (see Chapter 3), where there is too little insulin, or the insulin is released too slowly to cope with the amount of sugar that is released into the blood after eating. Anything that slows down the release of sugar from food will help to control the blood sugar level, because it will reduce the demand for insulin. If sugar is released over a longer period of time in smaller amounts, a small supply of insulin may be sufficient to the task. This sort of diabetes can often be controlled with a very high-fibre, high-starch, low-fat diet.

But can a low-fibre diet cause diabetes? Comparisons of people in different countries suggest that diabetes is linked with a western, and in particular an urban, diet. There is a high incidence of diabetes in almost all urban populations and even in the developing world there is higher prevalence among people living in urban centres than among the rural population. For example, the New Zealand Maoris have a lower incidence of diabetes than the white New Zealanders. Urbanisation tends to bring fairly profound changes in diet, in particular more refined carbohydrate and sugars, less fibre and more fat. But all these changes tend also to mean that the amount of overweight increases and in itself this would be likely to cause an increased incidence of diabetes (see Chapter 3).

In conclusion, there does seem to be a link between fibre, starch and diabetes, but the link seems to be with the control of existing diabetes. If fibre plays a part in the development of diabetes, it may be that people eating a low-fibre diet also tend to eat too many calories and are likely to be overweight. If a high-fibre diet can help to protect against the development of overweight, then it may also help to protect against the development of diabetes.

Bowel cancer

Scientists believe that bowel cancer develops in response to specific chemicals in the faeces. They do not know, however, whether diet, and in particular fibre, affects the number and type of such chemicals and/or creates the conditions under which they can cause a cancer to develop.

The suggestion is that fibre protects against bowel cancer, but there is as yet little evidence available to support the theory that bowel cancer is partially caused by a low-fibre diet. An understanding of the way fibre works in the body suggests that it is reasonable to suppose there is some sort of link. There are three reasons why a low-fibre diet might affect the risk of developing bowel cancer:

- a low-fibre diet results in small, hard stools which contain a higher concentration of whatever carcinogenic chemicals are present in the faeces; the large, bulky stools associated with a higher-fibre diet, containing lots of water, will have a lower concentration
- if any carcinogens are produced by the bacteria in the faeces, the slow transit time of low-fibre faeces gives them more time in contact with the bowel walls. Also, a longer transit time would mean there would be time for more carcinogens to be produced
- a low-fibre diet tends to be high in energy and fat and, in general, high energy intakes seem to make animal tissues more sensitive to carcinogens of all sorts and to large bowel cancer in particular.

Despite this commonsensical explanation of how fibre might have an effect, only one study has provided evidence for the theory that high intakes of dietary fibre protect against bowel cancer: urban Danes have four times the incidence of bowel cancer that the Finns have, and the Danes eat more white bread, less wholemeal bread, and fewer potatoes. Overall, the Danes in the study in question ate an average of only 17.2 grams of fibre a day while the Finns ate an average of 30.9 grams a day.

People who have bowel cancer do seem likely to have had lower fibre intakes in the past, though this sort of back-dated evidence is notoriously unreliable. In one study in Israel, bowel cancer patients reported lower intakes of high-fibre foods and no differences in their intakes of other types of food. Two other studies have suggested that bowel cancer patients have tended to eat fewer vegetables, but this may be an indication of the protective effect of Vitamins A and C (see Chapter 2).

Despite the lack of hard evidence, there remains a strong statistical link between bowel cancer and aspects of diet – there certainly seems to be an environmental element in the development of bowel cancer. The incidence of cancer of the colon varies by as much as 20 times in different parts of the world, generally being higher in more wealthy countries and lower in the poorer, developing world. A high incidence of bowel cancer is associated with relatively high intakes of meat, fat, sugar, eggs and energy (or calories) and with low intakes of cereals and pulses. There is very little international information about dietary fibre intakes so it has not been possible to compare incidences of fibre and bowel cancer direct.

There are many possible explanations for the apparent relationship between the western diet and bowel cancer – it could be the fat or the energy content of the diet that has the greatest effect, for example. In a sense, it is of no real significance to the general public which aspect of diet is having an effect, since a fibre-rich diet will almost inevitably also be one that is lower in fat, cholesterol and animal protein, and high in Vitamins C and A. This means that provided there is at least some link between diet and bowel cancer, a high-fibre diet would tend to protect against bowel cancer even if it isn't the fibre itself that helps.

Coronary heart disease (CHD)

The risk of developing CHD is primarily related to the amount of fat in the diet (see Chapter 4), but there is some evidence to suggest that other aspects of the western diet also have a part to play. In particular, a low-fibre diet might also have an effect on the risk of developing heart disease, possibly because of its effect on overweight and insulin production (see Overweight, above).

People who are overweight have an increased risk of developing CHD. A 10 per cent increase in body weight among men aged 35 to 44 is accompanied by a 38 per cent increase in CHD risk, and a 20 per cent increase among the same group is accompanied by an 86 per cent increase in CHD risk.

A low-fibre diet can result in the over-production of insulin (again, see Overweight, above) and this may be a factor in the development of atherosclerosis. Interestingly, diabetics have a high risk of developing CHD, but this could be because until recently diabetics were being advised to follow a low-carbohydrate diet in which a high proportion of calories would be likely to be gained from fat. A high-fat diet would be likely to increase the risks of developing CHD, independently of any fibre effect.

Research has failed to show any coherent pattern to links between fibre intake and CHD. Blood cholesterol levels can sometimes be lowered when men are put on a high-fibre diet, and this is particularly evident with soluble fibre (found in oats, fruit and vegetables and pulses). But the fibre intakes must be very high and the treatment works only in people with very high blood cholesterol levels. This makes it difficult to know what the effect of smaller amounts might be on more moderate blood cholesterol levels. In short, fibre does seem to have some effect on the synthesis of cholesterol, but since a high-fibre diet is usually also low in fat, it could be this that is having the effect.

Gallstones

The most common type of gallstones are cholesterol-based (see Chapter 3), so any substance which reduces the solubility of cholesterol in the bile may protect against gallstones, while any substance which increases the solubility of cholesterol in the bile may make gallstones more likely. The question, then, is whether the amount of fibre in the diet can affect the solubility of cholesterol in the bile.

The saturation of bile (saturated with cholesterol and thus likely to result in gallstones) can be reduced when people eat large amounts of bran. But experiments which showed this were done with women who already had saturated bile; in similar work among young men with unsaturated bile there was no such effect.

It seems likely that a high-fibre diet can affect the make-up of bile itself. Bile is composed of bile acids, phospholipids and cholesterol. In the bowel certain substances are reabsorbed into the body for future use; this happens in particular to certain bile acids. There is evidence to show that fibre can have an effect on the type of various bile acids that are reabsorbed and excreted, and so may have an effect on the cholesterol concentration of the bile.

It is certainly true that wild animals, who generally have a high-fibre diet, rarely develop gallstones. But gallstones can be induced by feeding them diets that are based on processed foods and are also low in fibre. In one study with rabbits, the gallstones then dissolved when they were fed a normal, high-fibre diet.

In general, gallstones are much more likely to occur in urban, industrialised societies; they are rare in the developing world, particularly in rural areas. One study of several urban areas in industrialised countries showed that there has also been an increase in incidence among young people and men, who are generally at lower risk than women and the elderly. All this tends to suggest that there is something about the western diet that is associated with an increased risk of gallstones, but whether it is excess calories, fat or fibre intakes, or all of these is not clear.

Tooth decay

The evidence that a high-sucrose, low-fibre diet is associated with a high incidence of dental decay is almost indisputable (see Chapter 7). It is not so clear what role, if any, fibre plays in preventing decay. All we know is that fibre has a number of effects which may help to protect against tooth decay.

For example, fibre alters the consistency of many foods, in general making them less sticky. White bread and flour stick to the teeth far more readily than do their wholemeal equivalents. Foods that require more chewing are also more thoroughly removed from the mouth and high-fibre foods take a lot more chewing than fibre-depleted equivalents. Chewing also stimulates the production of larger amounts of saliva than is normal, which helps to clear the mouth and act against the effect of any acid made as a result of bacteria feeding on sugars on the teeth.

6
TOO MUCH SALT?

Salt is a crucial ingredient in most people's diet. Once used to preserve food, it is now more likely to be used to bring out the flavour. Our palates are used to the taste of salt in food; many of us add it without thinking. If we stop to consider, we are likely to say that food without salt is tasteless or bland. Surprisingly, the average Briton gets most of their salt not from the salt-shaker but from bread, meat products such as pies and cold meats, breakfast cereals, cheese and fat spreads.

We know that on average, people in Britain eat at least 20 times as much salt as they need to keep the body ticking over, but is our dependence on salt causing health problems? It has been suggested that the amount of salt in the diet could be a factor in the development of high blood pressure and ultimately in stroke because of its association with high blood pressure. There have also been some suggestions that salt plays a part in the development of gastric cancer.

High blood pressure

High blood pressure is a very common condition in the UK and most of the rest of the western world. In Britain everyone's blood pressure rises with age and one in eight people has high blood pressure, while in communities with a more ethnic lifestyle and diet, for example some groups of Australian Aborigines and Greenland Eskimos, blood pressure problems are unheard of. Japan has a particularly high incidence of high blood pressure, and much of the evidence for a link with salt comes from studies of Japanese people.

Everyone's blood pressure varies according to the demands that are being made on their body, but some people's blood pressure is consistently at a higher level. Normal blood pressure is generally defined as giving a reading of 120/80. High blood pressure is determined by the pressure in the heart between contractions (that's the second figure – 80); with a reading of 90 someone is taken to have mild high blood pressure, at over 120 they are said to have severe high blood pressure. (For more on high blood pressure, see Chapter 3.)

Since the beginning of the century there has been an increasing amount of evidence suggesting some sort of link between salt and high blood pressure. But the link is not a straightforward one; although most countries with a high salt intake (such as Britain) also have a high incidence of high blood pressure, groups of British people with particularly high salt intakes are no more likely to have high blood pressure than their compatriots with lower salt intakes, and some people who have particularly high intakes don't appear to have any blood pressure problems at all.

This apparently contradictory evidence could be explained if everyone in a country like Britain had a sufficiently high salt intake to affect their blood pressure, and if having a higher than average salt intake didn't cause blood pressure to rise even higher. The fact that some people don't seem to be affected by high salt intakes might be explained if each individual's response is a matter not just of how much salt they eat but is also related to some inherited susceptibility to the effects of salt. There is some evidence to show that all these things might be true, but it is clear that if there is a relationship between salt and high blood pressure it is not a direct one.

As if this weren't complicated enough, more recent evidence from America suggests that high blood pressure could have as much to do with potassium and calcium intakes as it has to do with salt (or more properly sodium) intakes. This most recent evidence is still being hotly debated, and is discussed on page 100. But even the standard evidence for a relationship between salt and high blood pressure is still the subject of furious discussion among experts, so first, a detailed look at that.

The higher the salt intake, the higher the blood pressure

In the west, blood pressure tends to rise with age, so it would be easy to assume that increasing pressure is an inevitable part of the ageing process. Among rural people in the developing world however, blood pressure remains fairly constant with age. This suggests that there is some difference between the two types of society that is responsible for the difference in the incidence of blood pressure.

Various studies in different countries have looked at the relationship between salt and blood pressure levels and all have found that the higher the average salt intake, the higher the groups' average blood pressure levels (see Diagram 1). Studies which have looked at the incidence of high blood pressure or deaths from stroke in relation to salt intakes have also shown that there seems to be an association. For example, people in a part of Japan with higher sodium intakes than the Japanese average tended to have blood pressure of a higher level, and a higher incidence of hypertension and stroke than a group of Japanese who had lower sodium intakes, but whose environment was otherwise very similar.

In 1978 the results of a new study which looked at the relationship between sodium intakes and blood pressure levels in 52 centres around the world were reported. The results showed that there was an association between sodium levels and the incidence of high blood pressure taken across all the centres, although there were a number of anomalies. This study also showed a strong association between alcohol intake, body weight and blood pressure levels. In fact, these statistical links were much stronger than that with salt.

Today it would be thought unethical deliberately to introduce sodium to the diet of communities with otherwise low sodium intakes in order to see what effect this had on their blood pressure levels. In the early part of the century, though, several studies observed the introduction of salt to the diets of certain ethnic groups in the developing world, in particular, Indians in Panama, Chinese mountain people and Australian Aborigines. As salt intakes increased, so did the incidence of hypertension.

The thesis that sodium and hypertension are linked is lent weight by studies which have looked at people who have migrated. In particular, the Japanese, who generally have a very high sodium diet, have a significantly reduced incidence of hypertension and stroke when they move to countries like America, where salt intakes are comparatively much lower.

Some people with high salt intakes have normal blood pressure

The major failing in the theory that salt intakes and blood pressure are related is that were there a link, it would be reasonable to assume that individuals with high salt intakes would have higher blood pressures than individuals with low salt intakes. But comparisons of individuals' salt intakes and blood pressure levels have not produced convincing results; some studies have shown an association, others have not.

In 1984 a study of over 20,000 Americans, called the National Health and Nutrition Examination Survey (NHANES), reported the evidence from a sample of over 10,000 none of whom had special diets and none of whom was being treated for hypertension. The study showed that those with the highest blood pressure had the lowest sodium intakes and vice versa, quite the reverse of what might be expected. On the face of it, it looks as if this evidence rules out the sodium link, but there is a reasonably convincing explanation for the apparent contradiction.

The average American has a salt intake that is far in excess of human requirements and is also above the levels thought to be effective for maintaining normal blood pressure. For example, it is estimated that humans need a minimum of 500 –700 milligrams of salt a day, yet most people in this study had levels of between 1,600 and 5,000 milligrams. In other words, the majority of Americans have a high sodium intake and the fact that only some people develop high blood pressure might then be explained by the theory that some people are genetically susceptible or are salt-sensitive.

Genetic susceptibility might explain why comparisons between countries show a link between salt and blood pressure, but comparisons within countries often don't – there will be people in every population who have this susceptibility, so when different countries are compared, the genetic influence is balanced out. Within a single country, there may be relatively little variation between people's intakes and genetic susceptibility may obscure the influence of any other factor, such as sodium. But this theory wouldn't explain why the NHANES study concluded that the higher the blood pressure the lower the sodium intake and vice versa. The answer to this may lie in something else the study showed (see Not just a question of salt, below).

Are some people more susceptible than others?

Most of the evidence for some genetic role in the development of hypertension comes from work on rats done in the 1960s by a scientist called Dahl. He gave his rats a high-sodium diet and found that on average their blood pressure rose. But when he looked at individual rats he found a much more complicated picture: some rats' blood pressure rose over a long time, while in others the rise was very quick; while some rats' blood pressure rose a great deal, others showed only a mild increase; and a small number of rats maintained a perfectly normal blood pressure level despite high sodium intakes. This erratic or inconsistent response to increases in the amount of salt mirrors the picture in humans.

Dahl explained the varied response by identifying differences in the genetic make-up of the rats. He bred them and developed a strain of rats that he called 'salt-sensitive' – when their salt intakes were increased they all had a rise in blood pressure – and a 'resistant' strain – none of whom developed high blood pressure despite high intakes of salt. When kidneys were transplanted from resistant into salt-sensitive rats, their blood pressure fell, which tends to suggest that the susceptibility of some rats is a result of some built-in weakness in the kidneys.

Can we apply the findings of the rat study to human beings? Do some people develop high blood pressure and others not, because some people have kidneys that are better able to deal with high salt intakes than others? Hypertension does tend to run in families, and some studies in humans have shown that some individuals are more sensitive to the effects of sodium than others. There is also increasing evidence from laboratory work to show that cells from people with high blood pressure handle sodium differently to cells from people with normal blood pressure.

Even in susceptible individuals it may be that high blood pressure develops only if salt intakes have been high from birth, or at particularly crucial periods of life, for example during childhood. A study of 1,000 US Air Force men showed that those who had developed high blood pressure by the age of 48 generally had higher levels of blood pressure at 24 or so years old. Another study suggests that blood pressure levels from as early as one year old, give an indication of blood pressure levels in later life.

Reducing salt intakes can reduce high blood pressure

Reducing sodium intakes can lower blood pressure in people who already have hypertension. At the most extreme, diets with almost no salt content at all have been used to control very severe hypertension since the early 1920s. But such low salt levels could be achieved only in a controlled environment like a hospital and are not recommended for general adoption. The question then is, whether more moderate alterations in sodium intake have any effect on mild or moderate degrees of hypertension, as well as the more severe levels.

There is conflicting evidence, but studies tend to suggest that reducing salt intakes to about half the normal average level may have some effect on moderate hypertension, although no one is yet sure about its effect on mild hypertension. When exactly the same study was repeated on two groups of mild hypertensives, one group's blood pressure was lowered, but salt reduction had no effect on the blood pressure of the second group. The only difference between the two groups was that the group that showed a positive result had slightly higher blood pressure levels before the study than the group which showed no change.

Can lower salt intakes prevent high blood pressure?

Even if reducing salt intakes could be shown to bring down blood pressure in hypertensives, that doesn't necessarily mean that sodium intakes were the original cause of their problem, nor that low salt intakes will prevent people from developing high blood pressure. There have been very few studies in which whole communities have been asked to change their sodium intake and blood pressure has been monitored, and the studies that have been done are inconclusive.

In Japan and Belgium there were Government campaigns during the late 1960s and 1970s to encourage a reduction in salt intake. In Belgium, average salt intakes dropped from 15 grams a day to only 9 grams, between 1968 and 1981; there was a corresponding fall in deaths from stroke. In Japan, salt consumption shifted from 14.5 grams to 12.5 grams between 1971 and 1981 and in the same period there was a fall in the incidence of high blood pressure and deaths from stroke. But whether or not the salt reductions played any part in these health improvements is impossible to say, because so many other environmental influences are likely to have changed for individuals during this period: other aspects of diet; changes in the stresses related to working; smoking habits, and so on.

Not just a question of salt

The NHANES study concluded that the higher people's blood pressure, the lower their potassium and calcium intakes and also the reverse, that the lower their blood pressure, the higher their potassium and calcium intakes. Other studies have also pointed to some correlation between high blood pressure and low potassium intakes, and links have been found between potassium intakes and the incidence of hypertension and stroke. This is perhaps hardly surprising, since high sodium and low potassium intakes tend to go hand in hand in diet. There is very little sodium in raw foods, while potassium is found in relatively large amounts in raw fruit and vegetables, and just as sodium is added in the cooking and processing of food, potassium tends to be lost in these preparations.

If potassium does play a part in hypertension it may be particularly important in young people; one study showed that there were specifically low potassium intakes (as opposed to high sodium intakes) in a group of young hypertensives. There is also some evidence to show that increasing potassium intakes can reduce the incidence of hypertension in people who already have high sodium intakes. Rat studies lend some weight to this theory; feeding potassium in large amounts to salt-sensitive rats on a high-sodium diet and reduces their hypertension.

It could be that the balance of sodium and potassium is all-important, not the absolute levels of either mineral. Sodium and potassium need to be kept in balance for the fluid content inside and outside the body cells to be maintained. If salt intakes are increased and the body doesn't manage to get rid of the excess sodium, then the sodium/potassium balance may be upset. However, it may be that if the potassium levels are also raised, the balance can be restored. This would explain why in a country in which the majority of people have high sodium intakes (as in the NHANES study), potassium intakes rather than sodium intakes are a good indication of people who are likely to have high blood pressure.

A link between calcium and blood pressure has also been found in a number of other studies. But trials in which people with and without blood pressure problems were given calcium supplements of between one and two grams a day have shown varied results: blood pressure was reduced in people who had high blood pressure, but not in those with normal blood pressure; blood pressure was reduced more in people with high blood pressure; and blood pressure was reduced in only some people who had hypertension.

Studies on rats with normal blood pressure have shown that a calcium-free diet produces a rise in blood pressure, while in those with existing hypertension it causes a further rise in pressure. Conversely, a high-calcium diet helps to reduce a rise in blood pressure, even if the diet is also high in sodium. Importantly, calcium also plays a role in balancing sodium and potassium and the fluid levels in and outside the body cells, so the action of the three minerals is evidently linked.

In conclusion, there are a number of studies which show some sort of link between salt intakes and high blood pressure and reasonable explanations for the fact that salt intakes don't appear to have the same effect on all people. The complicating and relatively new evidence for links between potassium and calcium and blood pressure levels may prove significant – it may be that some complex balance of potassium, calcium and sodium is necessary for the maintenance of normal blood pressure. Debate between the experts is still vigorous, but it is not generally thought that reducing salt intake will do any harm and so taking precautionary action is generally thought to be a good idea, even in the absence of more compelling evidence.

Stomach cancer

Cancer of the stomach is not a particularly common form of cancer in Britain, but it is a serious and often fatal form of the disease. The incidence of stomach cancer seems to follow roughly the same world pattern as the incidence of hypertension and stroke; all three, for example, are very common in Japan. This has led some people to suggest that salt intake may also be linked to stomach cancer.

A study that looked at different regions in Japan, however, comparing the death rates for the two diseases with sodium intakes, showed that while there was a strong relationship between sodium intakes and the incidence of stroke, there was no such relationship between stomach cancer and salt intakes. They may be a link between salt intakes and cancer of the stomach, but at the moment there is far too little evidence available on which to base any recommendation.

7
TOO MUCH SUGAR?

In 1972 John Yudkin wrote a book called *Pure, White and Deadly* – the book was about sugar. Few people share his conviction that sugar is dangerous, but most of us think of sugar as bad for our teeth and our figures.

The average person in Britain eats 30 – 40kg of added sugar a year (see page 31 for a definition of added sugar), or 16 –22 teaspoonsful a day. It provides about 20 per cent of our calories, but that's all it offers in the way of nutrition. About two-thirds of this added sugar is put in foods by manufacturers and processors, most of it used simply to make products taste sweet, because we tend to like them that way – even small babies appear to have an untutored preference for sweet rather than savoury food, and young animals are no different.

Evidence suggests that it would be in the interests of our teeth to cut back the amount of sugar we eat and that reducing sugar intakes would also make it easier for many people to lose weight and maintain their new-found slimness.

Since a high sugar intake usually goes hand-in-hand with a low-fibre diet, many of the diseases that are thought to be related to low-fibre diets (see Chapter 5) also appear to be linked with high-sugar diets, for example gallstones, diabetes and cancer of the bowel. Although there is very little, if any, evidence that supports the theory that high sugar intakes play a direct part in the development of these diseases, making reductions might have an unsuspected benefit.

Tooth decay

Everyone knows that sugar is bad for teeth, or do they? You may not be surprised to know that the multi-million pound sugar industry disputes some of the evidence, but you might be taken aback to know that a handful of scientists also argue hotly about the primacy of sugar in the development of dental decay. It has been suggested that these experts are in the pay of the sugar industry, and specifically that many of them have received research grants. Would such funding matter? In a charitable mood one might suggest that the sugar industry chooses to fund certain scientists who are already sceptical about the evidence relating to the harm that sugar does. More cynically, one might suggest that scientists who receive funding are more likely to adopt a sympathetic approach to sugar in order not to lose financial backing from the industry.

In the final analysis, what is important is not why some scientists are sceptical about is the sugar/tooth decay link, but the fact that there are a few questions that need to be resolved. Although the case for a link between sugar and tooth decay is the strongest of all the relationships between disease and aspects of diet, there is still enough room for some people to claim that sugar is not the culprit and that we lay too much emphasis on it as the cause of decay. In particular, there is the question of whether starch is as bad for teeth as sugar and whether sugar in a refined form (what tends to be called 'added' sugar) is worse for your teeth than types of sugar that occur naturally in food – the glucose, fructose and lactose, for example, in fruit and milk. It appears that the sugar industry would have us believe that an apple is as potentially damaging to teeth, because of the natural sugars it contains, as a sugar lump, which is pure sucrose.

Is starch as bad as sugar?

The food we commonly call 'sugar' is sucrose. It can be white or brown, but it's all sucrose, processed from sugar cane and sugar beet. Fructose, glucose and lactose are sugars that are found naturally in foods like fruits and milk. These sugars can also be extracted and used to sweeten processed foods.

All starches and sugars can cause acid to be produced in the mouth. But less acid is found when starch is eaten, and all the evidence in humans shows that eating starchy foods is very unlikely to cause tooth decay. For example, people with high starch intakes and low sugar consumption tend to have low levels of decay and if refined sugars are introduced into the diet, decay levels rise. Even if starchy foods were found to contribute to tooth decay, the contribution is guaranteed to be small – sugars are much more likely to cause tooth decay.

Is refined sugar worse than natural sugar? Is fructose extracted from fruit worse for your teeth than fructose as part of a fruit? A comparison of the effects of sucrose, fructose extracted from fruit, and fruit containing fructose, showed that sucrose is more likely to cause decay than fructose when it is extracted from fruit, and extracted sugars (sucrose or fructose) are more likely to cause decay than the sugars eaten in fruits. In a Finnish study, people who had a normal diet containing sucrose had an average of 7.2 new instances of tooth decay, while those eating extracted fructose had only 3.8 new instances and those eating xylitol (a sweet-tasting substance that cannot cause decay) had no new decay at all.

Fruit juice is also more likely to cause decay than fruit, which suggests that if sugars are eaten in their natural state, bound up in the fibrous structure of the fruit, they are less likely to cause decay than sugars which are more readily available because the food is processed. It could also be that the chewing required to deal with high-fibre foods like fruit, stimulates an increased flow of saliva, which in turn protects the teeth against acid attack.

Some scientists have taken another line altogether, suggesting that sucrose is particularly harmful, not because it causes more acid to be produced, but because it encourages the growth of streptococcus mutans, a bacterium thought to be a particularly active cause of decay. Other sugars encourage the growth of less virulent types of bacteria.

In general, sugars are worse for teeth than starch, and refined or extracted sugar is more likely to cause decay than sugar in its natural state (in fruit for instance). It is not clear whether one type of sugar – sucrose, glucose or fructose – is worse than another. But ultimately, most experts point to sucrose simply because it is the sugar of which we eat the most. The foods that contain natural sugars, such as fruit, vegetables and milk, are too important a source of other nutrients to allow a recommendation that they be cut down because of the sugar they contribute to the diet.

How decay occurs

Although the role of sugar in decay is not in general disputed, it is worth looking at how the evidence has built up over the years. Some of the key pieces were collected in studies using psychiatric patients and prisoners, studies that today would be condemned as unethical. In terms of human rights it is clearly good that experiments like this are no longer permitted, but if they were, perhaps we would also have a clearer picture of the relationship between other aspects of diet and disease – fat and heart disease for example.

The theory of the relationship between sugar and decay is that plaque converts sugars to acid. The acids de-mineralise or soften the enamel on the tooth surface, which can result in decay (see Chapter 3).

There are two main planks to the fairly limited opposition to this theory: that various of the studies have flaws; and that more efficient ways to prevent tooth decay would be to stop plaque forming, by improving oral hygiene, and to strengthen the teeth against decay by using fluoride.

There is no doubt that some of the sugar studies are flawed, but there is such a wealth of evidence pointing in the same direction that finding a weakness in one or two studies cannot invalidate the whole picture. It is also true, in theory at least, that improving dental hygiene and/or strengthening tooth enamel could reduce the incidence of decay. But in practice, brushing your teeth can never prevent all decay. It takes only a tiny amount of plaque for decay to begin, and the most likely sites for decay are exactly those that are most difficult to clean: where two teeth meet, or in the tiny cracks on the surface of the back teeth. Tooth enamel can be strengthened with fluoride, but the most effective way to achieve this is by adding fluoride to the water supply, and there is considerable controversy about whether this represents an infringement of people's freedom. Fluoride toothpaste plays an important part in preventing decay but in the absence of more extensive fluoridation of drinking water, it makes sense to look to reduce decay by cutting back sugar intake as well.

Sugar and decay are linked

Average intakes of sucrose are related to the average incidence of tooth decay (see Table 1 – page 21 NACNE). In general, the incidence of decay is low among people who live on unrefined foods and relatively high in people who eat a lot of processed foods.

Also, people who have particularly high and low sugar intakes show correspondingly high and low incidences of tooth decay. For example, confectionery workers tend to have a higher incidence of dental decay than other factory workers. Studies in Israel and Japan have shown that the longer the workers had been in the sweets industry, the greater the differences became. In Japan, tooth decay is classified as an occupational disease for confectionery workers.

On the other hand, people with very low sugar intakes – for instance diabetics, who use a low-sugar diet to control their condition, Seventh Day Adventists, who have a very strict diet, and dentists' children – all have a lower than average incidence of tooth decay. The difference in decay rates when people are on a virtually sugar-free diet can be very striking. A study conducted in a South Australian children's home, Hopewood House, where the children had very little sugar, reported in 1963 that 46 per cent of the 12-year-old Hopewood children had no tooth decay, but the same was true of only one per cent of 12-year-olds in other schools in South Australia.

As sugar intakes increase, so does the incidence of decay. A study comparing teeth found in skulls from Anglo Saxon times with those of people living in 1957 found there had been a sevenfold increase in the incidence of tooth decay. Decay also appears to reduce as sugar intakes are lowered; in industrialised countries during wars, when sugar tends to be rationed, the incidence of decay decreased.

Not how much, but how often

If sugar is eaten as part of a meal it is not as harmful as if it is eaten alone, say between meals. In the 1950s over 400 inmates of a Swedish mental institution were fed extra sucrose. Some inmates were given the sucrose between meals in the form of chocolate, toffee or caramel, and others had their allowance with their meals. The group who ate their sucrose with meals had very little increase in tooth decay, but the group who ate sucrose in a sticky form between meals had a substantial increase in the incidence of decay.

Frequency of sugar consumption is important because it takes only a very little sugar to start the process of decay, and if a little sugar is eaten often enough, the teeth are constantly under attack from the acid produced by plaque. The effect on plaque of eating sugar can be gauged by measuring the pH level of the plaque before and after eating sugars; the lower the pH, the stronger the acid. The pH of plaque falls when sucrose and sugary snacks are eaten and the tooth enamel begins to soften when the pH falls to 5.5, or below. This level is reached within two to five minutes of rinsing the teeth in a sucrose solution. But it takes between 20 minutes and an hour for the pH to return to normal levels, so if further sugar is eaten or drunk, the pH remains low for longer.

If sugar is eaten on only a few occasions during the day there may be enough time for the tooth enamel to re-mineralise so that decay doesn't occur. The more frequently sugar is eaten, the more episodes of high acid production there are, and the more episodes of de-mineralisation occur.

The order in which foods are eaten can also affect the amount of acid that is produced and so have an impact on the likelihood of tooth decay. For example, if a meal ends with sweet foods, acid is produced by dental plaque unhindered, but if the sweet elements are followed by cheese, the alkali of the cheese can counteract the effects of the acid and the risk of decay can be reduced.

In general, there is considerable evidence that sugars cause dental decay, and that the likelihood of decay increases if sugars are eaten frequently and between meals. Although it is not clear that sucrose is any worse than other sugars, there are a number of reasons why, if you are cutting back on sugar, it is more sensible to cut back on sugars that are added to food in the manufacturing process, rather than sugars that are found naturally in other foods.

Overweight

Since most people gain between 14 and 16 per cent of their energy from sugars it seems reasonable to suppose that sugar might play some part in the development of overweight. It is an indisputable fact, however, that people who have very low sugar intakes can be fat and people who have very high sugar intakes can be slim. The most important factor in the development of overweight is how much energy people consume and how much they use. The form in which that energy comes is only of secondary importance.

It may be, however, that the nature of sugary and sweet foods encourages people to eat more of them than they need. Fibre-rich foods seem to have an effect on the type and amount of food that is eaten (see Chapter 5), so it seems reasonable to suggest that sugary foods also have an effect, if a different one. But, perhaps surprisingly, there is little real evidence to strengthen or weaken this theory.

People like sweet tastes. A study that rated reactions to different foods when people were hungry, showed that sweet foods were rated as more pleasant. Sweet and otherwise non-nutritious foods, such as confectionery, are not bulky and taste nice, so they can be eaten easily even after a large meal – they almost don't feel like food. And the fact that the sugar is hidden may also encourage over-eating: people are not aware of how much sugar they are consuming because it is not evident in some items, for instance soft drinks, some of which contain about 10 per cent of sugar by weight.

People choose the food that they eat for a whole host of reasons; physiological need is only one factor. It may be that sugary foods play a particular role in western societies that also encourages over-eating. Many people certainly think of sweet foods as a reward, comfort or treat.

Any food that can be eaten easily, even when people are not hungry and which has more energy value than people realise, is likely to be the cause of over-eating and so of obesity.

Undernutrition

High-sucrose foods may be a problem for another reason: if people eat an adequate but not excessive number of calories and a high proportion of sugary foods, it is quite possible that their nutrient intake will suffer. Many sweet foods provide a lot of calories, but very little in the way of other nutrients, which is why they are sometimes referred to as 'empty calories'. The people who are most vulnerable to this problem are the young, the old, and those who are dieting, all of whom tend to eat small amounts of food, from which they must gain the essential nutrients. The solution is to substitute foods such as bread, potatoes and fruit and vegetables for sugary foods, in order to maximise the intake of vitamins and minerals.

SECTION III

Action stations

8.

WHETHER TO CHANGE
YOUR DIET

Looking through the evidence for the relationship between various aspects of diet and health, helps explain why it is that the experts can't give a simple 'yes' or 'no' to the question of whether people in Britain should change their diet. In the absence of proof, some experts lean one way and some another, which often leaves consumers confused. So what should you do?

Does it make sense?

Changing your diet for the sake of your health but in the absence of concrete proof is an act of faith. Some of the evidence is more compelling than the rest, in particular the links between food and coronary heart disease, constipation, bowel cancer, overweight, high blood pressure and tooth decay. But there is no proof that people in general would benefit from a changed diet, and little evidence to show that any one individual would have better health as a consequence. Nor is there likely to be any.

Nonetheless, the evidence as a whole creates a fairly consistent picture – the standard high-fat, low-fibre, high-sugar and high-salt diet of the west is linked by a great deal of evidence to a range of disorders.

Often the evidence for the relationship between diet and a particular disease points to more than one link; for example, coronary heart disease is associated with high-fat and low-fibre diets. The truth is that a high-fat, high-sugar diet also tends to be low in fibre and is probably high in salt (simply because of its dependence on processed foods), while a low-fat diet is almost by definition a high-fibre and low-sugar diet.

Changing your diet in one respect will almost certainly result in other changes, which could have other benefits. A diet designed to reduce the risks of heart disease, for example, may also reduce the risks of bowel cancer or diabetes.

Increasingly the experts point to the balance of the diet as being important – the proportion of calories gained from fat as opposed to carbohydrate, and the proportion of carbohydrate that comes in the form of sugar, starch and fibre, for example. If changing one aspect of your diet means changing other aspects and one or other aspect is related to disease, there is a sense in which it doesn't matter to consumers whether it is the fat, fibre, sugar or salt in their diet that is the culprit. Why not just leave the scientists to thrash out the whys and wherefores?

Is it safe?

People who shouldn't change their diet

The recommendations for fat and fibre intake outlined here should not be applied to babies and children under the age of five. There are various reasons for this, but perhaps the most important is that very young children can't eat much food because their stomachs are small, and that means every bit of food must be made to count in terms of nutrient content. For example, a baby fed on skimmed milk would never be able to drink enough to get the calories it needed for growth.

People over the age of 60 also need to take care if they choose to follow the fat and fibre recommendations, because they too are likely to have low calorie intakes and must ensure they get sufficient vitamins and minerals. Pregnant women will benefit as much or as little as anyone else, but if they are making changes to their diet, they must take special care to ensure they are getting everything they need, especially vitamins and minerals.

People who should consult their doctor first

Anyone who already has diabetes, heart disease, high blood pressure, gallstones, diverticular disease or irritable bowel syndrome should consult their doctor before making radical changes to their diet, simply because changes may have to be made to any medications that are being taken. Some diabetics and hypertensives may be able to reduce the amount of any drug that they are currently taking, or even stop taking them altogether if they change their diet in an appropriate fashion. If your doctor hasn't already talked to you about the possible benefits of changing your diet, you might like to broach the subject yourself. Anyone who suffers from oedema (water retention such as menstrual swelling or swollen ankles), kidney disorders or a heart condition should check with their doctor before cutting back their salt intakes.

For the rest of us

No one has seriously suggested that the majority of people would do themselves any harm by changing their diet in the recommended direction, although a few questions have been raised about fat and fibre changes.

One concern is if people who already have a diet that is low in saturated fat, or who have a low blood cholesterol level, further reduce their saturated fat intake, they may increase their risk of developing some other disease or disorder. It is certainly true that, in some of the studies that have been done to try to reduce the risk factors for CHD, while CHD incidence has been reduced the participants have not lived any longer, but have died from some other cause. The other causes of death have varied enormously, however; no single cause appears to take over from CHD, so this concern seems to be unfounded.

You may also remember reading about 'muesli-belt malnutrition', a phrase coined by a doctor who claimed he had seen several children who were eating so much fibre that they weren't getting enough calories for their requirements – they were malnourished. Most doctors think there is no cause for concern, as long as children who have a high-fibre diet also have a varied one, and don't have excessive intakes of fibre. COMA and NACNE give a single fibre goal for everyone, but as discussed in Chapter 2, it may be that lower goals should be set for people with lower calorie intakes, including children. The fibre goals below are based on calorie intakes.

There are some people for whom making a decision to change diet is more straightforward because they are more likely to benefit – either they already have some condition like diabetes that the dietary changes can help them to control, or they are at particularly high risk of developing a disease. The best example of the latter is those at high risk of developing CHD, for whom changing their diet makes very good sense. People who are at high risk of developing CHD are those who currently smoke, don't exercise, are overweight and have a family history of the disease – generally speaking the more family members who have had CHD the greater your own risks. Of course, changing your diet can't outweigh the consequences of smoking, lack of exercise and overweight; these habits are also worth tackling.

An added bonus – more vitamins and minerals

One positive advantage of changing your diet is that your vitamin and mineral intakes are also likely to rise. The British Dietetic Association carried out a dietary study with 472 dietitians and their families. The participants were asked to complete a diary recording everything they ate and drank during a 'normal' week and then to try to alter their diets in line with NACNE guidelines for a further week, while keeping a second diary. The study showed that in general, vitamin and mineral intakes rose when the participants managed to alter their diets in line with recommendations, despite the fact that calorie intakes fell. If their calorie intakes had been maintained, their vitamin and mineral intakes would have risen still further.

However, there are two areas for concern about vitamin and mineral levels: intakes of calcium and zinc. A dietary study carried out by *Which?*, involving 28 members of the general public with little, if any, knowledge about nutrition, showed that not only were a significant number of the participants failing to get enough calcium before they changed their diets, but more of them failed to meet the requirement for calcium when they tried to change their diet in line with recommendations.

This may be because the study participants expressed a dislike for low-fat equivalents of full-fat dairy products, and many simply cut down dairy products to a minimum for the duration of the trial in order to meet the fat recommendations. Dairy products are our major source of calcium, but low-fat versions contain just as much calcium as their full-fat equivalents. This example serves to underline the need to add new foods to the diet as well as cutting back on existing intakes.

The second worry is that fibre contains a substance called phytate which can hinder the absorption of certain minerals, especially zinc. Cereal fibre, and in particular concentrated bran, contains a lot of phytate, and some nutritionists have expressed concern that a high-fibre intake might therefore lead to zinc deficiency. But it is generally thought that this could only affect people with particularly high requirements for zinc – children and pregnant women, for example – and only then if their zinc intakes were already low and their fibre intakes were exceptionally high.

Fewer calories – a good or a bad thing?

One potential effect of dietary change is that by cutting down fat and sugar, you are also likely to cut back calories. Both the *Which?* and the British Dietetic Association dietary studies showed that people tend to reduce their calorie intakes when changing their diet in line with recommendations. This could be seen as another bonus of changing your diet – a great many of us could do with losing a bit of weight. But no one can afford to lose weight indefinitely, and since the aim is to achieve long-term changes in your diet, you should replace the fat and sugar with more starchy carbohydrates like rice, pasta, bread and potatoes.

There are probably no risks attached to changing your diet, provided that you check with your doctor if need be (see above). Changing your diet may do you some good and it certainly won't do you any harm provided you act sensibly, following the guidelines given in Chapter 9.

If you think it makes sense to look at your diet in relation to health, the next practical step is to see how your diet compares with the current recommendations. The COMA and NACNE reports give guidelines for populations, so they are average 'goals' rather than recommendations for each individual. (If the goals were met, some people would be eating a lot more than the recommended levels and others would be eating less.) Nevertheless, it makes sense to use the population guidelines as the basis for setting individual goals. For one thing, they are all we have to go on. But COMA, in particular, recommends that individuals whose intakes are above the recommended fat levels should reduce them accordingly.

'But I've already changed my diet'

What consumers say . . .

With the media paying so much attention to food and health matters, it's easy to think that anyone who doesn't yet know about fat, fibre, sugar, salt and health must have been living the life of a hermit for the past ten years. In fact, although the majority of people have at least some idea of current dietary messages, there is a significant minority who are still unaware and many more are confused.

A survey carried out on behalf of Consumers' Association and others in 1985, asked 820 members of the general public whether they were aware of various nutritional terms and whether they thought intakes of these foods should be increased, reduced or maintained at about the same levels. While about eight out of ten people said fat and sugar should be cut down, and seven out of ten said the same about salt, only six out of ten thought fibre should be increased, and only around four out of ten thought that saturates should be reduced. It seems that despite the publicity, between three and four out of ten people have not yet got the message.

Table 14: Those who are aware of the term and said that people should . . .

Cut down		Increase		Eat same amount	
	%		%		%
Fat	83	Dietary fibre	62	Minerals	59
Sugars	79	Vitamins	61	Essential fats	50
Salt	69	Protein	58	Iron	49
Cholesterol	62	Energy	48	Sodium	41
Fatty acids	57	Iron	44	Carbohydrates	40
Calories	46			Energy	40
Saturates	39			Protein	36
Carbohydrates	38			Polyunsaturates	34

Consumer Attitudes to and Understanding of Nutrition Labelling, BMRB, 1985. Carried out on behalf of Consumers' Association, MAFF and the National Consumer Council

Of those who have heard recent dietary advice, a smaller proportion claim to be acting on it. For example, a survey of 2,014 people, carried out on 1987, asked 1,034 women whether they had altered their diets in any way in the last couple of years; 52 per cent of them claimed that they had made some changes in what they buy and eat, or give their families to eat, as compared with seven out of ten who thought too much fat was bad for health.

What we say and what we do are two potentially quite different things; many of those who claim to be acting according to dietary guidelines are not actually doing so. To follow dietary guidelines for fat, fibre, sugar and salt, people in general might be expected to: reduce their intakes of fatty meat and meat products, such as sausages, full-fat dairy products and fried foods; increase their intakes of fish and chicken; increase their fruit, vegetable and cereal intakes; switch from refined carbo-hydrates like white bread to unrefined carbohydrate, like whole-meal bread; stop adding sugar to tea and coffee; reduce their intakes of confectionery, soft drinks, cakes and biscuits, and stop adding salt to food when cooking, and at table.

In fact very few people claim to be making many of the

appropriate changes. For example, of 1,034 women questioned in the 1987 survey, only half claimed to have changed to wholemeal bread, or to be eating more of it and only 45 per cent claimed to be eating more salad, fruit and vegetables. Under two out of ten claimed that they were eating fewer dairy products, puddings and sweets, less red meat, and fewer fried foods (Table 15).

Table 15: Main changes to diet or purchase of food claimed by women

	%
Eat more/changed to wholemeal bread	50
Eat more salad/vegetables/fruit	45
Eat more fibre/bran	31
Eat less fat	27
Eat less sugar	23
Eat less salt	19
Eat fewer dairy products	17
Eat fewer food additives	16
Eat fewer puddings/sweets	16
Eat less red meat	16
Eat fewer fried foods	15

Survey of Consumer Attitudes to Food Additives, HMSO for MAFF, 1987

In general then, although about half the population claim to be making changes to their diets, there is no consistency to the sorts of changes that they claim to be making. One possible reason for this may be that people don't have enough information about the sorts of foods that they should be eating more and less of in order to follow the current dietary guidelines.

Insufficient information

A survey of 140 people, carried out by the Bradford Food Policy Research Group in 1985, asked what were the major sources of fat, fibre and sugar in the diet (see Table 16). The major sources

Table 16: Consumer views of the main sources of fat, fibre and sugar in the diet

Fat	% of respondents	Fibre	% of respondents	Sugar	% of respondents
Meat	71	Bread	76	Cakes	55
Butter	59	Cereals	61	Biscuits	46
Cheese	55	Vegetables	45	Confectionery	37
Milk	34	Fruit	30	Loose sugar	35
Margarine	20	Bran	20	Jam	14
Pastry	8	Baked beans	17	Tinned food	14
Cream	8	Potatoes	15	Cereals	13
		Pulses, rice, pasta	8	Fruit	11
		Porridge	6	Other	27
		Other	7		

Does the Consumer Really Care?, Stephen Fallows and Heather Gosden, Food Policy Research, University of Bradford, October 1985 of fat are meat, dairy products and oils and fats and most people in the survey seemed to realise this, although surprisingly few people identified milk and margarine as major sources. The major sources of sugar are packet sugar, cakes, biscuits, buns and pastries, soft drinks, confectionery and preserves. All these items featured toward the top of the respondents' list, but again relatively few people identified each major source. Similarly with fibre, of which the main sources are bread, flour, cereals and vegetables. In all cases, only one or two of the major sources of these nutrients were identified as such by more than half of the respondents, which suggests that there are deficiencies in the information available to the public about sources of fat, fibre, sugar and salt.

A survey of 761 members of the general public carried out for *Which?* in 1985 showed that people thought fibre was to be found in some very odd places: 52 per cent said they thought a portion of roast lamb contained either a little or a medium amount of fibre, while only 48 per cent said the same of an apple (see Table 17), whereas in fact roast lamb contains no fibre and an apple does.

Table 17: How much fibre in a portion of . . .

	None	Just a little	A medium amount
	% of respondents	% of respondents	% of respondents
Boiled egg	42	28	10
Roast lamb	23	31	21
Apple	18	24	24
Skimmed milk	51	22	7
Grilled bacon	29	33	16
Roast chicken	21	31	24
Chips	34	26	14
Beefburger	18	29	23
Smoked haddock	24	25	18

Marplan, for *Which?*, 1985

. . . and what consumers do

Despite the confusion and lack of information, there are a lot of consumers who know what the experts are saying, claim to be making changes in what they eat, and have sufficient information to do so sensibly. There should, therefore, be some quite significant changes in the national diet. However, this comforting picture doesn't stand up to scrutiny when you take a look at the sorts of food that are being bought by consumers.

One thing for which the National Food Survey is very useful, is showing trends in food consumption – whatever inaccuracies it may contain, they are the same each year and so it can give good information for comparisons between years. A comparison of the estimated intakes of selected foods in 1962 and 1985, shows that on average, the national diet was doing precisely the reverse of what the experts are advising (see Table 18). The only important change that went in line with expert recommendations was in butter and margarine consumption: butter went down by nearly half and margarine consumption went up.

Table 18: Changes in average consumption of selected foods from 1962 to 1985

Going up by	%	Going down by	%
Meat	3	Fresh fish	53
Margarine	37	Total fish	13
		Potatoes	19
		Fresh vegetables	28
		Fresh fruit	155
		Bread	29
		Cereals	20
		Butter	49

Household Food Consumption and Expenditure, HMSO for MAFF, 1986

Despite these somewhat depressing average figures, some shifts in consumption can be identified over the past four or five years which are more in line with expert recommendations. In particular, there has been a shift from full-fat to skimmed and semi-skimmed milks, from butter, lard and cooking fats to margarine, including low-fat spreads, and an increase in purchasing of fish, fresh and processed fruit and vegetables, fruit juices and breakfast cereals. Less bread is being bought, but more of it is wholemeal and brown and less is white, and less packet sugar is being bought (see Table 19).

Table 19: Comparison of food consumption in 1984 and 1986

Going up	1984	1986	Going down
	grams	*grams*	
	3.53	2.95	· Liquid full-fat milk
Low fat milk	0.33	0.70	
Total fish	4.89	5.16	
	2.87	2.27	Butter
Margarine	4.08	4.10	
	9.15	8.04	Sugar
Total vegetables	82.84	86.27	
Fresh fruit	18.99	20.33	
Fruit juices	5.28	6.84	
	20.05	16.54	White bread
Wholemeal bread	3.12	5.40	
Breakfast cereals	4.13	4.38	

Household Food Consumption and Expenditure, HMSO for MAFF, 1986

In theory at least, almost everyone in Britain has a diet that is too high in fat, particularly saturated fat, too low in fibre, and too high in salt and sugar. But in practice, some people may already have diets which are more or less like the guidelines in at least one or more respects. It's most unlikely that changing your diet would do you any harm, even if you already meet some of the goals, but since the COMA report refers to individuals who fail to meet the goals being the ones who need to change their diet, we have devised a questionnaire to help you assess your own intakes, see how they match up to the guidelines and decide what sort of level of change you would have to make to alter your diet to meet them.

The food intake questionnaire

The questionnaire that follows was devised in conjunction with the Nuffield Laboratories of Comparative Medicine at the Institute of Zoology in London, at Regent's Park Zoo. Forty-two people weighed and noted down in diaries everything they ate over seven days. Two weeks later they filled in a questionnaire giving information about the frequency with which they normally ate a range of foods. The diaries were analysed for nutritional content and the results for the diaries were compared with the results given by the completed questionnaires. The object of the exercise was to develop a questionnaire which gave a reasonable approximation to the figures given by keeping a diary.

To help you interpret your results, we have turned the COMA and NACNE guidelines into a more workable form, giving the number of grams of fat, saturated fat, fibre, sugar and salt to aim for. With the exception of the fibre goal, these are maximum levels; eating a bit less would do no harm. This is particularly the case with the goals for fat and saturated fat, which are based on recommended average calorie intakes – figures that we know are set too high for today's needs (see Chapter 2).

Why it's approximate

This questionnaire will help to give a reasonable indication of your dietary intakes, but any questionnaire of this sort involves making approximations. First, we ask only about foods that make a significant contribution to average intakes of fat, saturated fat, fibre, sugar and salt. If we have not listed a food it is because it generally makes only a small contribution to intakes, but if you eat a lot of it, this could throw your results off balance.

Secondly, no one has absolute recall of what they eat, and most people have very little idea of how much of each food they eat. It may help to keep a rough diary for a few days before filling in the questionnaire – recording what you eat and even weighing a few portions. But it is important that, when you fill in the questionnaire, you think not of the food eaten in the last few days, but of your diet in general. This necessarily involves some generalisation.

Finally, we have given scores for the contribution different foods make to nutrient intakes, but they are based on average portions. These have been assessed by MAFF on the basis of dietary studies, but you may eat particularly big or small portions.

The explanation of how to fill in the questionnaire is overleaf.

How to fill in the questionnaire

Decide roughly how many portions of the first food you eat in a week and fill in the box labelled 'number of portions'. Do this for the entire list given in the questionnaire.

Next, assess each nutrient in turn. Starting with fat, multiply the number of portions you eat by that food's gram score for fat and write the total in the next box. Do this for all the foods that contribute to fat overall.

Now add up the fat gram scores, using the total boxes at the end of each food section. Then turn to page 148 and check your intake against the daily intake goal.

Sometimes it has been necessary to list foods more than once. Camembert, for example, is a medium-fat cheese and as such is listed with Edam. Camembert is also, however, high in salt, and is listed again for salt content. When this occurs, it is important to give information for every entry, even though it may seem repetitious.

In Chapter 9 we give some ideas about the amounts of fat, fibre, salt and sugar in 100 grams of a variety of foods. You could use this to help you work out what sort of change is needed in your diet. For example, if you need to cut back by around 10 grams of fat or so, this might be achieved by changing to a lower fat milk and using a low-fat spread.

Food intake questionnaire: How much of these foods and their elements do you eat in a week?

Biscuits and cakes	Number of portions		Fat		Saturated fat		Salt		Added sugar		Fibre	
Sweet biscuits (eg one chocolate covered or sandwich)		×	3	=	2	=	1	=	3	=		
Plain, sweet biscuits (eg one digestive or rich tea)		×	2	=	1	=	1	=	2	=		
Cake, plain or jam sponge (one slice – 50g)		×	3	=	1	=	3	=	18	=		
Cake or bun, rich (eg one slice gateau, butter-iced, chocolate, cream – 75g)		×	16	=	8	=	5	=	26	=		
Other cakes or buns (eg one slice Madeira, gingerbread, one rock cake, one doughnut or Danish pastry) – 75g		×	3	=	5	=	7	=	11	=		
Crispbread, one		×									1	=
			TOTAL		TOTAL		TOTAL		TOTAL		TOTAL	

Dairy produce	Number of portions	Fat	Saturated fat	Salt	Added sugar	Fibre
Cheese, cream (eg Philadelphia) – 30g	☐ ×	☐ = 14	☐ = 9			
Cheese, full-fat (eg Stilton, Cheddar) – 40g	☐ ×	☐ = 13	☐ = 8			
Cheese, medium-fat (eg Edam, Camembert) – 40g	☐ ×	☐ = 9	☐ = 6			
Cheese reduced fat (eg Shape & Tendale) – 40g	☐ ×	☐ = 6	☐ = 4			
of which Cheese, high salt (eg blue, Camembert, processed and smoked) – 40g	☐ ×			☐ = 14		
Cheese, medium salt (eg Cheddar and other hard cheese, Edam) – 40g	☐ ×			☐ = 8		
Cheese, low salt (eg cottage, cream or curd) – 30g	☐ ×			☐ = 3		
Milk, whole (full-fat) – 140ml (¼ pint)	☐ ×	☐ = 5	☐ = 3	☐ = 1		

	Number of portions		Fat		Saturated fat		Salt		Added sugar		Fibre
Milk semi-skimmed – 140ml (¼ pint)		×	3	=	2	=	1	=			
Cream (one to two tablespoonfuls) – 45g		×	?	=	10	=					
Yoghurt, full-fat, natural or fruit (eg Greek/Smatana) – one small pot		×	15	=	9	=	1	=			
Yoghurt, full-fat, natural or fruit (eg Greek/Smetana) – one small pot		×	2	=	1	=	1	=			
of which Yoghurt, fruit or flavoured – one small pot		×							22	=	
				TOTAL		TOTAL		TOTAL		TOTAL		TOTAL

Eggs	Number of portions	Fat	Saturated fat	Salt	Added sugar	Fibre
Egg, boiled or poached – one egg	☐ ×	5 = ☐	2 = ☐	2 = ☐		
Egg, fried, scrambled or omelette – one egg:	☐ ×	11 = ☐				
of which fried in vegetable oil	☐ ×		3 = ☐	10 ☐		
fried in butter or lard	☐ ×		5 = ☐			
Quiche – one slice – 120g	☐ ×	34 = ☐	12 = ☐	15 = ☐		
		TOTAL ☐	TOTAL ☐	TOTAL ☐	TOTAL ☐	☐

Fat spread	Number of portions		Fat			Saturated fat			Salt			Added sugar	Fibre
Butter – 110g (¼lb)	□	×	91	=	□	59	=	□	25	=	□		
Low-fat margarine-type spread (eg Gold, Outline) – 110g (¼lb)	□	×	46	=	□	13	=	□	20	=	□		
Low-fat butter-type spread (eg Kerry Light) – 110g (¼lb)	□	×	46	=	□	29	=	□	20	=	□		
Margarine, high in polyunsaturates (eg sunflower, soya) – 110g (¼lb)	□	×	91	=	□	16	=	□	23	=	□		
Margarine, other soft – 110g (¼lb)	□	×	91	=	□	29	=	□	23	=	□		
Margarine, hard – 110g (¼lb)	□	×	91	=	□	40	=	□	23	=	□		
			TOTAL		□	TOTAL		□	TOTAL		□	TOTAL □	TOTAL □

Meat and meat products	Number of portions		Fat		Saturated fat		Salt		Added sugar	Fibre
Bacon – 2 rashers		×	9 =	☐	4 =	☐	18 =	☐		
Ham – one slice		×	5 =	☐	2 =	☐	9 =	☐		
Liver sausage/pâté – one sandwich covering – 40g		×	7 =	☐	3 =	☐	6 =	☐		
Other processed meats (eg salami, tongue) – one slice		×	7 =	☐	3 =	☐	7 =	☐		
Tinned and processed meats (eg corned beef, spam or salami, tongue) – one slice		×	6 =	☐	2 =	☐	8 =	☐		
Beefburgers – one small – 35g		×	6 =	☐	3 =	☐	8 =	☐		
Sausages – one large – 60g		×	13 =	☐	5 =	☐	16 =	☐		
Meat pies, heavy (eg individual steak & kidney pie) – 200g		×	47 =	☐	19 =	☐	32 =	☐		

Number of portions		Fat		Saturated fat		Salt		Added sugar	Fibre
Meat pies, medium (eg individual pork pie) – 140g	×	33	=	13	=	22	=		
Meat pies, light (eg one sausage roll) – 60g	×	14	=	6	=	9	=		
Meat and meat dishes, lean only – 280g	×	24	=	11	=				
Meat and meat dishes, lean and fat – 280g	×	54	=	25	=				
Chicken and chicken dishes, no skin – 140g	×	8	=	3	=				
Chicken and chicken dishes, meat and skin – 140g	×	20	=	6	=				
	TOTAL		TOTAL		TOTAL		TOTAL	TOTAL	

Fish	Number of portions		Fat	Saturated fat	Salt	Added sugar	Fibre
Oily (eg trout, mackerel) – one average sized fish	[ ]	×	14 = [ ]	3 = [ ]	2 = [ ]		
of which Smoked (eg mackerel) – one fish – 150g	[ ]	×			43 = [ ]		
Smoked salmon – 60g	[ ]	×			16 = [ ]		
Tinned (eg tuna, pilchards, sardines) – one sandwich filling portion – 50g	[ ]	×	6 = [ ]	? = [ ]	6 = [ ]		
Shellfish (eg cockles, mussels, prawns) – 40g	[ ]	×			18 = [ ]		
Roes, pâté, taramosalata – one portion as starter – 40g	[ ]	×	15 = [ ]	4 = [ ]	3 = [ ]		
White, fried (eg cod, haddock) – one steak or fillet – 110g	[ ]	×	13 = [ ]		5 = [ ]		

	Number of portions	Fat	Saturated fat	Salt	Added sugar	Fibre
of which fried in vegetable oil	× [ ]		2 = [ ]			
fried in butter or lard	× [ ]		5 = [ ]			
White, steamed, grilled – one steak or fillet – 80g	× [ ]	1 = [ ]		2 = [ ]		
		TOTAL [ ]	TOTAL [ ]	TOTAL [ ]	TOTAL [ ]	[ ]

Vegetables: Fresh, frozen or tinned	Number of portions	Fat	Saturated fat	Salt	Added sugar	Fibre
Green leafy, fresh (eg cabbage, spinach, broccoli) – 90g	□ ×					3 = □
Peas, beans, lentils and chick peas – 90g	□ ×					9 = □
of which Tinned with added salt	□ ×			7 = □		
Fried vegetables (other than potatoes, eg mushroom, onion) – two tablespoonfuls: fried in vegetable oil	□ ×	12 = □	2 = □			
fried in butter or lard	□ ×		7 = □			
Potatoes, chipped, roast, sautéed – 190g	□ ×	15 = □	2 = □			2 = □
fried in vegetable oil	□ ×					

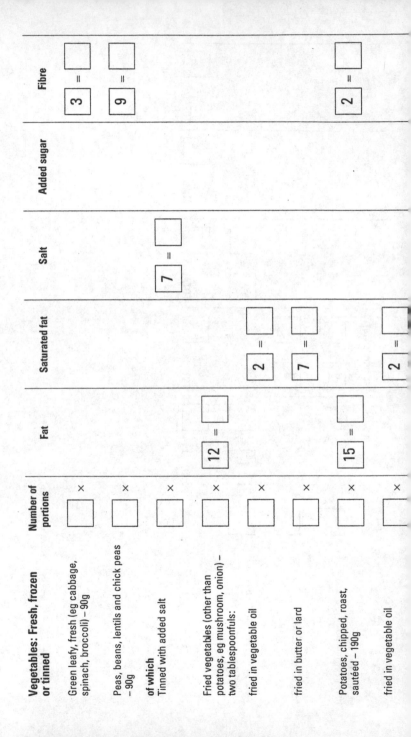

fried in butter or lard ☐ ×

Potatoes, boiled or baked – 180g ☐ ×

Salad (eg mixed salad including tomatoes) – 110g ☐ ×

Root, fresh (eg carrots, parsnips) – 60g ☐ ×

Other tinned vegetables

Baked beans – half a small tin – 135g ☐ ×

Tomatoes – 100g ☐ ×

Sweetcorn – 90g ☐ ×

of which tinned with added salt – 90g ☐ ×

$6 = $ ☐

$16 = $ ☐

$4 = $ ☐

$3 = $ ☐

$1 = $ ☐

$2 = $ ☐

$10 = $ ☐

$1 = $ ☐

$5 = $ ☐

TOTAL ☐   TOTAL ☐   TOTAL ☐   TOTAL ☐   TOTAL ☐

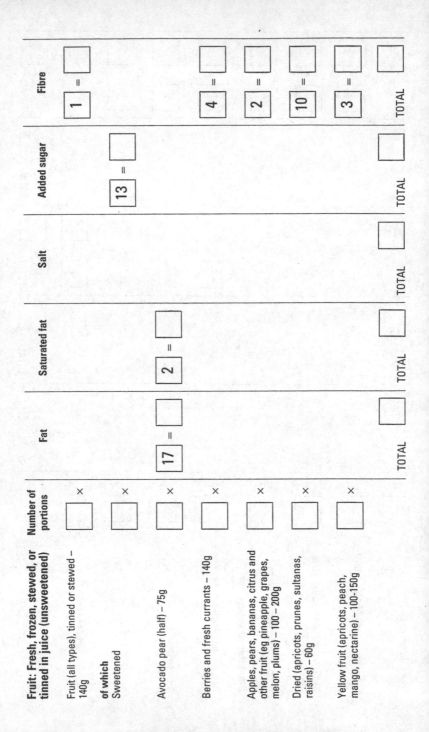

Fruit: Fresh, frozen, stewed, or tinned in juice (unsweetened)

	Number of portions	Fat	Saturated fat	Salt	Added sugar	Fibre
Fruit (all types), tinned or stewed – 140g	× □					1 = □
of which Sweetened	× □	17 = □			13 = □	
Avocado pear (half) – 75g	× □		2 = □			4 = □
Berries and fresh currants – 140g	× □					2 = □
Apples, pears, bananas, citrus and other fruit (eg pineapple, grapes, melon, plums) – 100 – 200g	× □					10 = □
Dried (apricots, prunes, sultanas, raisins) – 60g	× □					3 = □
Yellow fruit (apricots, peach, mango, nectarine) – 100-150g	× □					
		TOTAL □	TOTAL □	TOTAL □	TOTAL □	TOTAL □

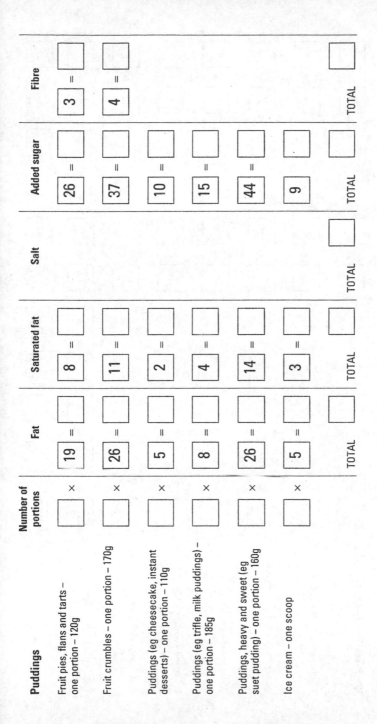

Puddings	Number of portions	Fat		Saturated fat		Salt	Added sugar		Fibre	
Fruit pies, flans and tarts – one portion – 120g	×	19 =	☐	8 =	☐		26 =	☐	3 =	☐
Fruit crumbles – one portion – 170g	×	26 =	☐	11 =	☐		37 =	☐	4 =	☐
Puddings (eg cheesecake, instant desserts) – one portion – 110g	×	5 =	☐	2 =	☐		10 =	☐		
Puddings (eg trifle, milk puddings) – one portion – 185g	×	8 =	☐	4 =	☐		15 =	☐		
Puddings, heavy and sweet (eg suet pudding) – one portion – 160g	×	26 =	☐	14 =	☐		44 =	☐		
Ice cream – one scoop	×	5 =	☐	3 =	☐		9	☐		
		TOTAL	☐	TOTAL	☐	TOTAL ☐	TOTAL	☐	TOTAL	☐

Bread and rolls	Number of portions	Fat	Saturated fat	Salt	Added sugar	Fibre
Wholemeal bread – one slice – 35g	× [ ]			5 = [ ]		3 = [ ]
Wholemeal roll – one roll – 45g	× [ ]			6 = [ ]		4 = [ ]
Brown, 'Granary-style' bread – one slice – 35g	× [ ]			5 = [ ]		2 = [ ]
White bread – one slice – 30g	× [ ]			4 = [ ]		1 = [ ]
White roll – one roll – 45g	× [ ]			6 = [ ]		1 = [ ]
Pitta – one small – 75g	× [ ]			10 = [ ]		3 = [ ]
Pizza – one small – 200g	× [ ]	23 = [ ]	10 = [ ]	17 = [ ]		4 = [ ]
		TOTAL [ ]	TOTAL [ ]	TOTAL [ ]	TOTAL [ ]	TOTAL [ ]

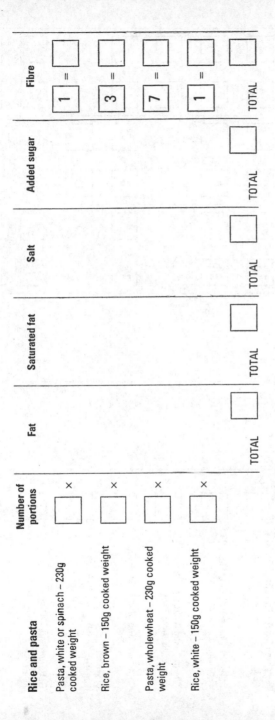

Rice and pasta	Number of portions	Fat	Saturated fat	Salt	Added sugar	Fibre
Pasta, white or spinach – 230g cooked weight	☐ ×					1 = ☐
Rice, brown – 150g cooked weight	☐ ×					3 = ☐
Pasta, wholewheat – 230g cooked weight	☐ ×					7 = ☐
Rice, white – 150g cooked weight	☐ ×					1 = ☐
		TOTAL ☐	TOTAL ☐	TOTAL ☐	TOTAL ☐	TOTAL ☐

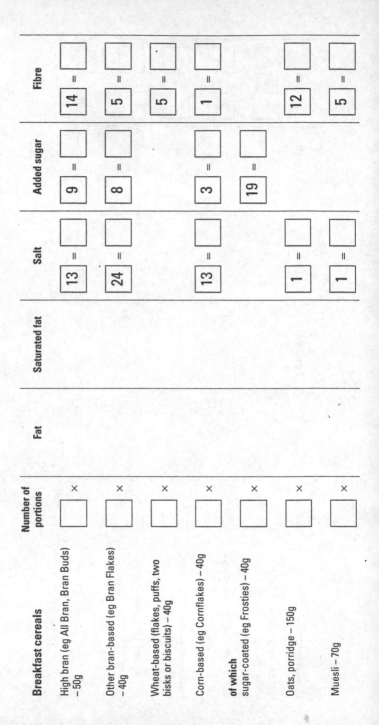

Breakfast cereals	Number of portions	Fat	Saturated fat	Salt	Added sugar	Fibre
High bran (eg All Bran, Bran Buds) – 50g	[ ] ×			13 = [ ]	9 = [ ]	14 = [ ]
Other bran-based (eg Bran Flakes) – 40g	[ ] ×			24 = [ ]	8 = [ ]	5 = [ ]
Wheat-based (flakes, puffs, two bisks or biscuits) – 40g	[ ] ×					5 = [ ]
Corn-based (eg Cornflakes) – 40g	[ ] ×			13 = [ ]	3 = [ ]	1 = [ ]
of which sugar-coated (eg Frosties) – 40g	[ ] ×				19 = [ ]	
Oats, porridge – 150g	[ ] ×			1 = [ ]		12 = [ ]
Muesli – 70g	[ ] ×			1 = [ ]		5 = [ ]

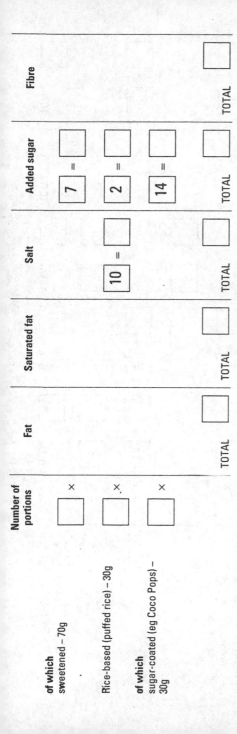

Number of portions	Fat	Saturated fat	Salt	Added sugar	Fibre
of which sweetened – 70g □ ×				7 = □	
Rice-based (puffed rice) – 30g □ ×			10 = □	2 = □	
of which sugar-coated (eg Coco Pops) – 30g □ ×				14 = □	
	□ TOTAL	□ TOTAL	□ TOTAL	□ TOTAL	□ TOTAL

Snacks	Number of portions	Fat	Saturated fat	Salt	Added sugar	Fibre
Peanuts, one medium bag – 40g	☐ ×	20 = ☐	4 = ☐			3 = ☐
of which Salted peanuts, one medium bag – 40g	☐ ×			4 = ☐		
Crisps and other potato and cereal deep-fried snack foods, one medium pack – 35g **of which** salted	☐ × ☐ ×	13 = ☐	4 = ☐	5 = ☐		4 = ☐
Other nuts (unsalted) – 40g	☐ ×	19 = ☐	2 = ☐			1 = ☐
Olives, five olives – 15g	☐ ×	1 = ☐		7 = ☐		
		TOTAL ☐	TOTAL ☐	TOTAL ☐	TOTAL ☐	TOTAL ☐

Confectionery: Chocolate, toffee and chocolate-covered bars

	Number of portions	Fat		Saturated fat		Salt	Added sugar		Fibre
Large and heavy (eg Mars, Yorkie, Yorkie, Fruit'n Nut) – 70g	□ ×	17 =	□	10 =	□		39 =	□	□
Large and light (eg four-bar KitKat, Twix, Topic, Aero) – 50g	□ ×	12 =	□	7 =	□		28 =	□	
Small and light (eg Crunchy, Flake, Smarties, Treets, two-bar KitKat, Wispa, four chocolates or toffees) – 35g	□ ×	8 =	□	5 =	□		20 =	□	
Muesli bars – 30g	□ ×	5 =	□	1 =	□		4 =	□	4 = □
Sweets, boiled, mints, chews, pastilles and gums – one tube/pack – 35g	□ ×						25 =	□	
		TOTAL □		TOTAL □		TOTAL □	TOTAL □		TOTAL □

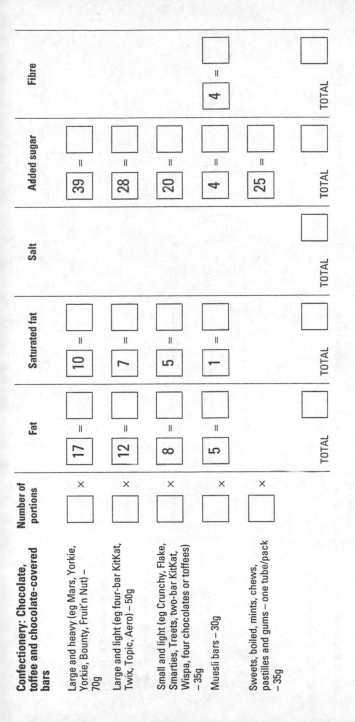

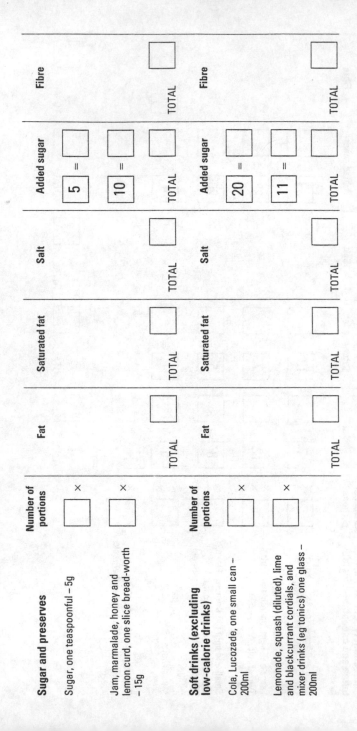

Sugar and preserves

	Number of portions	Fat	Saturated fat	Salt	Added sugar	Fibre
Sugar, one teaspoonful – 5g	☐ ×				5 = ☐	
Jam, marmalade, honey and lemon curd, one slice bread-worth – 15g	☐ ×				10 = ☐	
		TOTAL ☐	TOTAL ☐	TOTAL ☐	TOTAL ☐	TOTAL ☐

Soft drinks (excluding low-calorie drinks)

	Number of portions	Fat	Saturated fat	Salt	Added sugar	Fibre
Cola, Lucozade, one small can – 200ml	☐ ×				20 = ☐	
Lemonade, squash (diluted), lime and blackcurrant cordials, and mixer drinks (eg tonics) one glass – 200ml	☐ ×				11 = ☐	
		TOTAL ☐	TOTAL ☐	TOTAL ☐	TOTAL ☐	TOTAL ☐

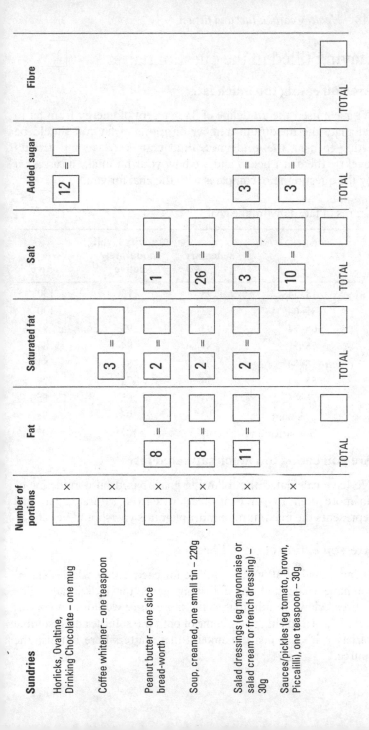

Sundries	Number of portions	Fat	Saturated fat	Salt	Added sugar	Fibre
Horlicks, Ovaltine, Drinking Chocolate – one mug	[ ] ×				[ ] = 12	
Coffee whitener – one teaspoon	[ ] ×		[ ] = 3			
Peanut butter – one slice bread-worth	[ ] ×	[ ] = 8	[ ] = 2	[ ] = 1		
Soup, creamed, one small tin – 220g	[ ] ×	[ ] = 8	[ ] = 2	[ ] = 26		
Salad dressings (eg mayonnaise or salad cream or french dressing) – 30g	[ ] ×	[ ] = 11	[ ] = 2	[ ] = 3	[ ] = 3	
Sauces/pickles (eg tomato, brown, Piccalilli), one teaspoon – 30g	[ ] ×			[ ] = 10	[ ] = 3	
		TOTAL [ ]	TOTAL [ ]	TOTAL [ ]	TOTAL [ ]	TOTAL [ ]

Having filled in the questionnaire. . .

Are you eating too much fat?

We have used the guideline of 35 per cent of energy from fat to calculate the maximum number of grams of fat you should be eating to meet the guidelines. Find your sex, age and activity level on the chart below and see how your fat intake as assessed by the questionnaire compares with the goal for you.

Grams of fat, daily intake goal:

	Age	sedentary	Activity level: moderately active	very active
Men	18–34	98	113	130
	35–64	93	107	130
	65–74	93	93	93
	75+	84	84	84
Women	18–54	84	84	84
	55–74	74	74	74
	75+	65	65	65
	pregnant	93	93	93
	breast-feeding	107	107	107

Are you eating too much saturated fat?

We have calculated the following goals based on a guideline of no more than 15 per cent of calories from saturated fat; this represents the maximum number of grams you should be eating.

Are you eating enough fibre?

Using a goal of 10 grams of fibre for each 1,000 calories eaten, we have calculated the following goals for individuals. The figures below are minima; eating more fibre would do no harm, but it's worth trying to eat some of both the soluble and insoluble variety – it's not just the amount that matters here but also the source.

Grams of saturated fat, daily intake goal:

	Age	sedentary	Activity level: moderately active	very active
Men	18–34	36	41	48
	35–64	34	39	48
	65–74	34	34	34
	75+	31	31	31
Women	18–54	31	31	36
	55–74	27	27	27
	75+	24	24	24
	pregnant	34	34	34
	breast-feeding	39	39	39

Grams of fibre, daily intake goal:

	Age	sedentary	Activity level: moderately active	very active
Men	18–34	25	29	34
	35–64	24	28	34
	65–74	24	24	24
	75+	22	22	22
Women	18–54	22	22	22
	55–74	19	19	19
	75+	17	17	17
	pregnant	24	24	24
	breast-feeding	28	28	28

Are you eating too much sugar?

NACNE and COMA say cut back from an average 104 grams total sugars (78 grams of which is 'added') to 96 grams total sugars (no more than 70 grams of which is added). If 20 per cent of calories come from sugar, at least 75 per cent of this is added sugar and a 10 per cent reduction is recommended, the following individual goals can be calculated.

Grams of added sugar, daily intake goal:

	Age	sedentary	Activity level: moderately active	very active
Men	18–34	90	104	121
	35– 64	86	99	121
	65–74	86	86	86
	75+	77	77	77
Women	18–54	77	77	77
	55–74	68	68	68
	75+	60	60	60
	pregnant	86	86	86
	breast-feeding	99	99	99

Are you eating too much salt?

The goal for salt is much more straightforward, a single figure for everyone – a target of 9 grams a day, based on a population goal of a 10 per cent reduction of current intake. To convert your questionnaire score for salt into grams, divide by 10. A score of 112, for example, equals 11.2 grams.

Finally, are you overweight?

You may be surprised by our height/weight chart opposite, because it doesn't make any allowances for sex and it appears to be very generous about the acceptable weights. The chart is based on statistics that show the points at which weight affects people's risks of dying as a result of ill health. These statistics don't point to any differences between men and women of the same height and weight.

Acceptable weight: Your weight won't adversely affect your health. If you think you're overweight, exercise is probably the answer to tone you up.

Overweight: Your increased risk of ill health is only very slight, but the risk of your continuing to put weight on and gradually edge into the very overweight or obese categories is ever increasing. Controlling your weight is now a priority to stop any further increases.

Very overweight: You run an increased risk of developing CHD, hypertension, diabetes, gallstones, arthritis and even some forms of cancer. You should definitely try to lose weight, but you should probably ask your doctor's advice first.

Obese: You should already be receiving advice from your doctor since your weight will be a major handicap. If not, make an appointment to discuss the problem.

Diagram 7: Are you overweight?

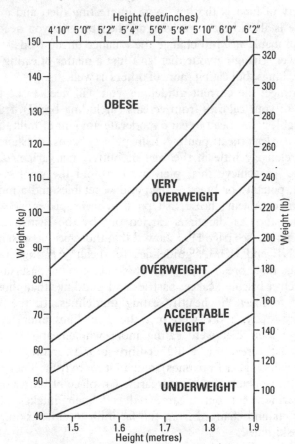

9
HOW TO CHANGE

The four ground rules for starting a healthy eating programme are:

1. Don't cut anything right out of your diet
Variety of food is the key to an interesting diet, and a varied intake is also likely to provide all the nutrients you need. You will probably need to change the balance of the foods you eat, however; changing your diet isn't just a matter of eating less of some things, but eating more of others as well.

To meet the current guidelines you will need to be getting most of your calories from cereals (including bread), fruit and vegetables; you need to eat a moderate amount of milk, cheese, yoghurt, lean meat, poultry, fish, pulses, beans, nuts and eggs; and relatively little in the way of butter, margarine, oils and sugar. To achieve this, plan meals round the staples – rice, pasta, potatoes or bread – then add vegetables and a moderate amount of protein (cheese, fish, poultry, beans, pulses and so on).

The study of dietitians carried out by the British Dietetic Association (see page 115) showed that those people who met the NACNE and COMA guidelines for healthy eating ate more cereals, more bread (especially wholemeal), more pasta and rice, and fewer biscuits, cakes, pastries and puddings than those who failed to meet the healthy eating guidelines. In the *Which?* dietary study, those who met the guidelines after trying to change their diet were eating more wholemeal bread, more breakfast cereal (or a higher-fibre brand), more vegetables (especially higher fibre ones), and a lot more fruit. They also ate a high-in-polyunsaturate margarine (in place of butter or other margarine), cut out cream, reduced their intakes of meat products and changed from full-fat milk to either skimmed or semi-skimmed.

You can make a lot of headway simply by swapping one version of a food for another: choose a high-fibre cereal instead of a low-fibre one, or a low-fat spread instead of a full-fat one, for example. This way you don't need to change too much what you eat, nor how you cook it, only what you buy. This is by far the easiest way to start to change your diet, and food manufacturers and retailers have done a lot to help by bringing out new versions of foods: baked beans with reduced sugar and salt, for instance. Also, adapt your favourite recipes: use yoghurt instead of cream, low-fat milk instead of full-fat milk.

2. Try out new foods and different cooking methods
Healthy eating does not have to be boring, nor do you have to become a vegetarian or a 'crank', but it does help if you are prepared to experiment with ingredients and cooking techniques. For example, when you cut back on red meat, make sure you get protein from some other source: pulses and beans, cheese and eggs are all good sources of protein, as are fish and poultry. Most people learn how to cook by watching at home, and because 'old-style' eating has predominated in Britain many of us feel comfortable cooking meat but are less certain what to do with a pile of fresh vegetables. Buying a new cookery book can be a good spur. Try some different approaches to cooking – some Eastern dishes are high in fibre and low in fat, and there are an increasing number of interesting vegetarian cookbooks around.

3. Don't make life a misery
You don't need to completely eliminate your favourite foods, just cut down on the amount you eat and the frequency with which you have them. The aim is to change the overall balance of your diet, and that means you can still eat some high-fat, high-sugar, high-salt and low-fibre foods. If you've decided to change your diet, the plan is to change for life, and no one wants to be miserable for life.

4. Don't go too far too quickly
Be realistic. You are more likely to be successful if you take a step at a time, than if you wake up one Monday morning having

decided to give up everything that's 'bad' and eat everything that's 'good'. The chances are that come Thursday, you'll be craving your favourite 'bad' food and be in danger of abandoning all your good intentions.

OUT SHOPPING
New foods for old

Cutting down fat

- Buy skimmed or semi-skimmed milk in place of full-fat, silver-topped milk.
- Buy yoghurt (preferably low-fat), in place of cream. Even a switch from double to single cream will reduce your fat intake.
- Try a low-fat spread on bread, and a high-in-polyunsaturate margarine for baking and cooking.
- Look for low-fat alternatives for dairy products in general: for example, low-fat yoghurts, low-fat fromage frais and quark and lower-fat cheeses (see What's in food, below).
- Choose a high-in-polyunsaturate oil (see What's in food) for cooking and dressings.
- Buy fewer meat products.
- Buy lean red meat – beef and lamb – and more fish and poultry.
- Buy pulses and grains to replace some meat. If you haven't the time to soak and cook pulses, look for ready-cooked tinned varieties.
- Choose lower-fat biscuits and cakes, and try making your own with high-in-polyunsaturated fats.
- Generally look for low-fat foods – salad dressings and mayonnaise, low-fat sausages and so on.

Boosting fibre intake

- Buy more bread (whatever the variety) and switch from white to brown, and preferably to wholemeal whenever possible.
- Choose wholewheat flour in place of white.
- Buy more rice and pasta, and especially wholewheat pasta and brown rice.

- Choose wholegrain wheat and bran breakfast cereals (see What's in food, below).
- Select lots of fresh and frozen fruit and vegetables.
- Buy dried fruits and unsalted nuts in place of sweets and other snack foods.
- Buy more pulses. Most supermarkets now have a selection of cooked pulses in tins, not just baked beans.
- Buy wholemeal oat and bran biscuits (sweet and savoury) and look out for wholemeal crispbreads.

Reducing sugar intake
- Replace chocolates and sweets with fresh and dried fruits and nuts.
- Try not to buy much packet sugar, but if cutting out added sugar is unpalatable, try one of the artificial sweeteners instead.
- Look for low-calorie soft drinks and fruit juice in place of standard soft drinks – lemonade, mixers and colas, for example.
- Choose unsweetened fruit juice.
- Select fruit tinned in fruit juice rather than syrup.
- Buy natural yoghurt and add your own chopped fruit, rather than buying sweetened fruit yoghurts.
- Buy fewer cakes and biscuits, and buy plainer ones – digestives and fruit biscuits rather than of chocolate, cream-filled and iced.
- Select reduced-sugar jams.
- Opt for breakfast cereals with less sugar (see What's in food).
- Look for lower-sugar versions of savoury foods – low-sugar baked beans and soups, for example.

Cutting down salt
- Buy less cheese (especially blue cheeses and processed varieties). Buy small amounts of strong-tasting cheese, so you use less.
- Buy fewer of the highly salted snack foods, like peanuts and crisps.

- Reduce the amount of smoked and pickled fish and meats you buy and don't choose foods packaged in brine.
- Don't buy smoked bacon.
- Buy fewer meat products – sausages, pies and cooked meats.
- Cut down on sauces and pickles, but stock up on herbs and spices to cook with.
- Choose an unsalted butter or low-salt spread.
- Buy fresh and frozen vegetables instead of tinned. If you have to buy tinned, look for low-salt varieties.
- Find a lower-salt breakfast cereal (see What's in food, below).
- If you can't get used to food cooked without salt, try one of the low-salt or salt-substitute products. They tend to have a slightly more bitter taste. Salt substitutes contain potassium chloride, which can be dangerous for people with kidney conditions, so these people should take their doctor's advice first.
- Look for low-salt versions of processed foods – tomato and vegetable soups with a low sodium content, for example.
- Buy fresh fruit and vegetables that are potassium-rich, for example: apples, bananas, apricots, dates, grapefruit, oranges, prunes, raisins, beans, Brussels sprouts, cabbage, sweetcorn, peas, peppers, potatoes, radishes.

Watch the labels

Labels on food can help you make a selection, but they can also mislead you, especially in the area of nutrition and health.

In a survey carried out for Consumers' Association, the National Consumer Council and MAFF in 1985, nine out of ten people said that they would find helpful nutrition labelling that gave fat, fibre, sugar and salt contents. In July 1987 the Government issued a set of guidelines for food manufacturers and retailers to follow when labelling their foods with nutrition information, and recommended listing one of the following:

1. energy, protein, carbohydrate and fat content
2. energy, protein, carbohydrate and fat content with a breakdown to show saturates

3. energy, protein, and carbohydrate content, with a breakdown to show sugars; and fat content with a breakdown to show saturates, sodium and fibre.

The guidelines are entirely voluntary at the moment, so some foods may carry labels that conform to them, others have labels of an altogether different form, and some labels give no information at all. In a survey of 422 food items carried out for *Which?* in 1988, only 15 items had labelling that fulfilled recommendation 3, above, and 107 items had no nutrition information whatsoever.

The Government plans to introduce regulations to ensure that if food manufacturers and retailers choose to give nutrition information, they will have to follow one of the three formats in the guidelines, but they do not plan to make labelling compulsory. This will make it impossible for consumers to compare information on similar products and choose accordingly. Even if all manufacturers did choose to give at least some information on their products, the labels would not necessarily be comparable because one might use the first form of the nutrition label and another the second or third form. Only the third version of this label includes all the information that consumers need to follow experts' recommendations about healthy eating.

An increasing number of products also now carry general claims relating to their nutritional content: 'high-fibre', 'low-fat', 'reduced sodium', 'no added sugar' and so on. The problem is that as yet there are no regulations to control the use of these claims, and different manufacturers may use the same words to mean different things. For example, research for a *Which?* report in August 1988 showed that when the Co-op says on a label 'low-fat' it means the product has less than 3 grams of fat in every 100 grams, but Sainsbury uses the same term to mean 'this food has no more than 50 per cent of the fat of a similar product'.

Evidently, consumers are being confused, and arguably misled, by these sorts of claims. A survey of 1,328 people conducted for the *Which?* report showed that nearly half of them thought that a cereal that made a 'high-fibre' claim contained more fibre than one that made no such claim. This is not necessarily the case. The Government currently considering regulations to control claims of this sort and to ensure that when such claims are made, the product packaging also carries a full nutrition label (the fullest of the three versions above), so consumers can see what else the food contains – it could be high in fibre, but it may also be high in salt.

The new market for foods to fit in with healthy eating guidelines has also led to a rash of claims for foods and their ingredients being 'natural'. In the same survey for *Which?*, seven out of ten people wrongly thought that a product carrying the label '100% natural' could not contain any additives and eight out of ten people thought the food was likely to be healthy. In fact there is no reason why 'natural' should necessarily also mean 'healthy'. The Government also has plans to control the use of claims like this.

IN THE KITCHEN

Cutting down fats

- Cut all the visible fat off meat.
- Eat smaller portions of leaner meat.
- Don't add fat when roasting. Baste with water or meat juices as they emerge, or try pot roasting (with a little liquid and the lid on).
- Drain off fat during and after cooking.
- Leave cooked meat and stews to cool, so that fat solidifies, and take off the fat layer before re-heating.
- Grill meat and meat products on a rack, rather than frying them, to allow fat to drip out into grill pan.
- Don't eat the skin on poultry.
- Use pastry as little as possible – make single-crust pies, or substitute potato or oaty toppings instead.
- Spread less butter or margarine on your bread.
- If you make chips, cut them thickly and fry them in very hot oil, preferably one that is high in mono- or polyunsaturates.

Thin chips or crinkle-cut varieties soak up more fat, because they have a larger surface area. Also, the hotter the fat the sooner the surface of the chip is sealed and the less fat it soaks up.

- Instead of oily salad dressings, try making dressings based on yoghurt and lemon juice, with caraway seeds, fresh mint and other herbs for extra flavour.
- Use skimmed and semi-skimmed milk when cooking. The chances are that no one will know the difference, although they might notice it in their tea or on cereal.
- Use yoghurt in recipes instead of cream.
- Use fresh herbs in place of butter on fresh vegetables, and steam vegetables for extra flavour.
- Use a little of a strongly flavoured cheese.
- Steam fish and poultry to avoid fats in cooking, or cook fish in foil parcels, with no extra fat.
- Stir-fry food in the Chinese style – it uses very little fat.
- If you have a microwave oven, use it as much as possible – microwave cooking requires very little fat.
- Use a non-stick pan whenever you are frying, so you need to use virtually no fat.
- In general, grill, bake, steam, poach, casserole and boil instead of frying and roasting foods.

Boosting fibre intake
- Use wholewheat flour in cooking and baking, even as the thickening for sauces.
- Cook fruit and vegetables in their skins (having scrubbed them well), and eat the skin – this is the highest-fibre part of the food.
- Try stuffed and baked vegetables as a main dish.
- Use rice and pasta in puddings as well as hot dishes.
- Make rice- and grain-based puddings – semolina, tapioca and rice pudding, for example.
- Use flaked cereals, such as rolled oats, as a crunchy topping for fruit and savoury crumbles.
- Cut bread more thickly.

Reducing sugar intake
- In recipes for cakes and biscuits, try using half the sugar suggested. If the results are not to your liking, add a little more sugar until you find the right level for your taste – it's often a lot less than recommended.
- Try cooking with artificial sweeteners if you can't stomach baked foods, for instance cakes, with less sugar.
- Use alternative flavourings in cooking, for instance dried fruit, or spices, for example cinnamon.
- When you do eat particularly sweet foods, eat them as part of a meal, have them only about once a day and try to follow them with something that will reduce the effect of any acid that is produced in your mouth – eat some cheese or yoghurt afterwards, for example.
- Stop putting sugar in tea and coffee, or wean yourself off it gradually.
- Make fruit and milk puddings with no added sugar.
- Spread honey, jam and marmalade a little thinner, or use a savoury spread like peanut butter.

Cutting down salt
- Always taste your food before adding salt – you may be surprised to find it doesn't need it. One study showed that 60 out of 100 people salted their food at the table and 45 of these did so before even tasting it.
- Invest in a salt shaker with very small holes. The same study showed that people shake the salt pot for the same amount of time irrespective of how much salt is coming out; the smaller the holes the less salt they were adding to their food.
- Try reducing the amount of salt that you use in cooking, until you find a minimum level that suits you.
- Use herbs and spices for extra flavour.
- Don't use salt when cooking vegetables – it reduces their potassium content. Steam vegetables instead, to maximise the flavour.
- Use home-made stocks and vegetable cooking water with herbs and spices, in place of salty stock cubes.

What's in food

Some examples of the fat, fibre, sugar and salt contents of some foods that make significant contributions to fat, fibre, sugar and salt intakes.

FAT CONTENT

Milk
Grams of fat in each 100 grams
Full-cream (gold top) 4.8g (14g in ½ pint)
Full-fat (silver or red top) 3.8g (11g in ½ pint)
Semi-skimmed (red and silver striped top) 2g (5.5g in ½ pint)
Skimmed (blue and silver striped top) 0.1g (0.3g in ½ pint)

Cheese
Grams of fat in each 100 grams
High-fat:
(eg Stilton, Cheddar-type, cream) 30–50g
    cream cheese 47g
    Stilton 40g
    Cheddar 33g
Medium-fat:
(eg Edam, processed, Camembert) 20–25g
    Brie and Camembert 27g
    Edam 25g
    processed 25g
Reduced-fat: Cheddar-type 17g
Low-fat:
(eg cottage or curd) 0.4–4g
    cottage 4g

**Yoghurt, cream and
ice-cream**

Grams of fat in each 100 grams
Yoghurt: full-fat natural   4g
    low-fat natural   1g
Cream: single   21g
    whipping   35g
    double   48g
Ice-cream: non-dairy   8g

**Spreads and
cooking
fats and oils**

Grams of fat in each 100 grams
Total fats:
    lard, dripping and all the oils   100g
    Butter and all the margarines   80g
Saturated fats
High-in-saturates:
    lard, butter, block margarine, palm
    and coconut oils   30–55g saturates
Medium-in-saturates:
    soft margarine and nut oil   20 – 30g
    saturates
Low-in-saturates:
    low-fat spreads,
    pure vegetable oils and
    polyunsaturated margarines   5–20g
    saturates

Potatoes

Grams of fat in each 100 grams
Deep-fried chips   11–19g
Oven chips   6g
Roast potatoes   5g
Boiled and baked potatoes   0.1g

Meat/fish

Grams of fat in each 100 grams
Beef, roast sirloin, lean and fat   21g
Beef, roast sirloin, lean only   9g
Lamb, roast leg, lean and fat   18g

Lamb, roast leg, lean only 7g
Pork, roast leg, lean and fat 20g
Pork, roast leg, lean only 7g
Chicken, roast with skin 14g
Chicken, roast without skin 5g
Corned beef 12g
Pork sausages, grilled 32g
Pork pie, individual 27g
Sausage roll 36g
Grilled lean bacon 19g
Fried lean bacon 22g
Fish paste 10g
Oily fish (eg mackerel) 12g
Deep-fried cod 10g
Steamed cod 1g

	Grams of fat in each 100 grams
Cakes, biscuits, pastry and snacks	Madeira cake 17g
	Digestive biscuits 21g
	Chocolate cake 27g
	Shortcrust pastry 32g
	Potato crisps 36g
	Roasted peanuts 49g

FIBRE CONTENT
(By Southgate method – see page 34)

	Grams of fibre in each 100 grams
Bread	Wholemeal 8.5g
	Malted wheat grain (eg 'Granary') 6g
	Bran-enriched white 5.7g
	Brown 5.1g
	White 2.7g

Flour

Grams of fibre in each 100 grams
Wholemeal   9.5g
White   3g

Breakfast cereal

Grams of fibre in each 100 grams
Bran-based   25g
Wheat flakes and biscuits   12g
Wheat biscuits   13g
Muesli-type, oat and crunchy   7g
Porridge   0.8g
Puffed rice and cornflakes   7g

Branded cereals

Grams of fibre in each 100 grams
All-Bran   30g
Bran Buds   28g
Bran Flakes   17g
Coco Pops   1g
Cornflakes   3.4g
Crunchy Nut Corn Flakes   1.6g
Farmhouse Bran   18g
Frosties   1.2g
Fruit'n'Fibre   10.1g
Grapenuts   6.2g
Honey Smacks   4.6g
Muesli, Swiss-style   8.1g
   with extra fruit   5.4g
   with no added sugar   11.1g
Nutri-Grain   12.4g
Puffed Wheat   8.8g
Ready Brek   6.8g
Rice Krispies   1.1g
Ricicles   0.9g
Shredded Wheat   10.1g
Shreddies   10.9g
Special K   2.7g
Start   9.3g

Sugar Puffs   4.8g
Sultana Bran   15.5g
Weetabix   8.5g
Weetaflake   11.6g
Weetaflake'n'raisin   7.2g
Weetos   11.7g

Rice and pasta (raw weight)

Grams of fibre in each 100 grams
Wholewheat pasta   11.5g
White pasta   5.1g
Brown rice   3.8g
White rice   2.7g

Vegetables

Grams of fibre in each 100 grams
Spinach   6g
Sweetcorn kernels   6g
Green leafy vegetables: broccoli, green
    beans   3g
Root vegetables: carrots, parsnips,
    swedes   3g
Salad and other watery vegetables:
    lettuce, cucumber   up to 2g
Potatoes: baked with skin   2g
             chipped   1g
             boiled or mashed   1g

Fruit

Grams of fibre in each 100 grams
Dried fruit   17g
Nuts   9g
Fresh fruit: apple, banana, orange
    2.5g
Orange   2g
Banana   3.5g
Soft fruit: strawberries, apricots   2g

Pulses

Grams of fibre in each 100 grams
Lentils, kidney beans, butter beans
   (cooked weight) 6g
Lentils (dry weight) 12g
Kidney beans (raw) 25g
Baked beans 7g
Peas 12g

SUGAR CONTENT

Cakes and biscuits

Grams of sugar in each 100 grams
Fruit cake 43g
Iced chocolate cake 54g
Sponge cake, jam-filled 48g
Doughnut 15g
Jam tart 38g
Chocolate digestive 30g
Plain digestive 16.5g
Ginger nut 33g

Drinks

Grams of sugar in each 100 grams
Cola 10.5g
Diet cola none
Lemonade 5.5g
Orange squash (diluted) 6g
Blackcurrant juice drink (diluted) 10g
Tonic water 8.5g
Drinking chocolate (4.5g in each
   teaspoon) 74g

Puddings

Grams of sugar in each 100 grams
Ice cream 20–23g
Fruit yoghurt 18g
Diet fruit yoghurt 7.5g
Natural yoghurt 6.5g

Fruit pie　15g
Canned fruit in syrup　25g
Canned fruit in juice　12.5g
Apple crumble　24g
Jelly　14g
Trifle　19g
Rice pudding　9g

Breakfast cereals

Grams of sugar in each 100 grams
Bran-based　14–20g
Puffed rice　10g
Chocolate flavoured puffed rice　37g
Muesli　26g
Shredded wheat　0.4g
Cornflakes　8g
Sugar-coated cornflakes　40g
Wheat biscuits　6g
Bran-based and dried fruit　25g
Wheat puffs　1.5g
Sugar-coated wheat puffs　35–37g

Branded cereals

Grams of sugar in each 100 grams
All-Bran　15.4g
Bran Buds　25.7g
Bran Flakes　19g
Coco Pops　38.2g
Cornflakes　7.2g
Crunchy Nut Corn Flakes　36.3g
Farmhouse Bran　23.1g
Frosties　41.5g
Fruit'n'Fibre　26.7g
Grapenuts　12.1g
Honey Smacks　39.2g
Muesli, Swiss-style　23.7g
　with extra fruit　22.3g
　'with no added sugar'　15.3g

Nutri-Grain   8.4g
Puffed Wheat   0.3g
Ready Brek   1.7g
Rice Krispies   10.6g
Ricicles   39.8g
Shredded Wheat   0.8g
Shreddies   10.2g
Special K   18g
Start   31.5g
Sugar Puffs   56.5g
Coco Sultana Bran   32.9g
Weetabix   6.4g
Weetaflake   6.4g
Weetaflake'n'raisin   24.6g
Weetos   29.4g

Confectionery

Grams of sugar in each 100 grams
Milk chocolate   56.5g
Chocolate/caramel bar   54–56g
Peppermints   100g
Boiled sweets   87g
Liquorice sweets   67g

Spreads

Grams of sugar in each 100 grams
Chocolate spread, jam, honey,
    marmalade   66g
Reduced-sugar jams   33g

Sauces and pickles

Grams of sugar in each 100 grams
Sweet pickle (1 dessert spoon = 6.5g)
    33g
Tomato ketchup, brown sauce
    (1 tablespoon = 4g)   23g

Savoury foods

Grams of sugar in each 100 grams
Tomato soup   6.5g
Baked beans   5.2g
Reduced-sugar baked beans   3g

---

and for comparison

Grams of sugar in each 100 grams
Apple juice   11.5g
Milk   4.7g
Banana   14.5g
Orange   8g
Dried apricots   43g

SALT CONTENT

Canned food

Grams of salt in each 100 grams
Baked beans   1.2g
Carrots   0.7g
Chickpeas   2.1g
Spaghetti in tomato sauce   1.2g

Snacks

Grams of salt in each 100 grams
Potato crisps   1.4g
Salted peanuts   1.1g
Olives in brine   5.6g

Bread

Grams of salt in each 100 grams
1.4g

Breakfast cereals

Grams of salt in each 100 grams
Bran flakes   1.6–2.5g
Cornflakes   2.5–3.3g
Oat cereals (porridge-type)   none
Rice-based   0.8–3.3g
Wheat biscuits   0.8–1.6g

Branded cereals

Grams of salt in each 100 grams

All-Bran   3.7g
Bran Buds   1.3g
Bran Flakes   2.3g
Coco Pops   2.2g
Cornflakes   2.8g
Crunchy Nut Corn Flakes   1.9g
Farmhouse Bran   2.2g
Frosties   1.9g
Fruit'n'Fibre   1.5g
Grapenuts   1.5g
Honey Smacks   0.8g
Muesli, Swiss-style   1g
   with extra fruit   0.3g
   'with no added sugar'   0.1g
Nutri-Grain   1.3g
Puffed Wheat   trace
Ready Brek   trace
Rice Krispies   3.2g
Ricicles   2.2g
Shredded Wheat   trace
Shreddies   1.4g
Special K   2.9g
Start   1g
Sugar Puffs   trace
Sultana Bran   1.5g
Weetabix   0.9g
Weetaflake   0.9g
Weetaflake'n'raisin   0.5g
Weetos   2g

Biscuits and cakes

Grams of salt in each 100 grams

Cream crackers   1.5g
Digestive   1.1g
Oatcakes   3g
Rock cakes   1.2g
Madeira cake   0.95g

Meat and meat products	*Grams of salt in each 100 grams*
	Meat and poultry 0.2g
	Bacon, raw 3.5g
	Gammon, raw 3g
	Gammon, grilled 5.7g
	Corned beef 2.4g
	Ham 3.1g
	Luncheon meat 2.6g
	Sausages, raw 2g
	Beefburger, raw 1.5g
	Pork pie 1.8g
	Stock cubes 25.8g

Sauces and pickles	*Grams of salt in each 100 grams*
	Brown sauce 2.5g
	French dressing 2.4g
	Piccalilli 3g
	Sweet pickle 4.3g
	Tomato ketchup 2.8g

Fish	*Grams of salt in each 100 grams*
	Cod 0.2g
	Mackerel 0.3g
	Kippers 2.5g
	Fish fingers 0.8g
	Shrimps 9.6g
	Prawns 4g

Soups, tinned	*Grams of salt in each 100 grams*
	1–1.2g

	Grams of salt in each 100 grams
Cheese	Camembert 3.5g
	Cheddar 1.5g
	Danish Blue 3.6g
	Edam 2.5g
	Parmesan 1.9g
	Stilton 2.9g
	Processed 3.4g

	Grams of salt in each 100 grams
Spreads	Butter, salted 2.2g
	Margarine and other spreads 2g
	Butter and margarine, unsalted trace

EATING OUT

In a restaurant

If you don't eat out very often or this is a special occasion, forget the guidelines – nothing you can eat in one meal can have a detrimental effect on your healthy eating plan. Even if you have sherry trifle with double cream, your average weekly intakes won't be raised by much. Only if eating out is a fairly regular event do you need to take a long hard look at the menu for foods that are reasonably consistent with your new eating plan.

If you do eat out a lot, then you may find it difficult, or boring to eat at the more 'traditional' restaurants, but here are some guidelines:

- for a starter, choose fruit or vegetable-based dishes with little sauce – melon instead of pâté, for example
- for a main course, select fish or chicken dishes without cream sauces, have a pasta dish or look for rice-based dishes. If you decide to have red meat, choose something lean and preferably without a sauce, and have it grilled, rather than fried. Order lots of vegetables and potatoes, preferably baked or steamed and not fried, sauté or chipped

• for pudding, select something fruit-based, without pastry, and don't have cream.

Take-aways

There's no getting away from the fact that take-aways are often convenient, but there's also no escaping the fact that they tend to be high in salt and fat and not very high in fibre. A survey carried out by the British Nutrition Foundation in 1985 showed that about one in three people said that they ate a take-away at least once a week, so these can play a significant role in some people's diets.

In September 1987 *Self Health* (now *Which? Way to Health*) asked a nutritionist to assess 14 commonly eaten take-away meals to see whether any of them fitted in with a healthy eating plan. One of the features of take-away food is that it is often fried, but nonetheless, *Self Health* managed to find some take-aways with a low fat or high fibre content, or a better balance of fat and fibre.

The take-aways given a 'healthier' rating were: a baked potato with cottage cheese filling; a beanburger in a wholemeal bun; chicken tandoori and chapati, dahl and boiled rice; doner kebab with salad; chicken chow-mein. (The last two were low in calories because the portions were small, which is one of the reasons they came out moderately well. Smaller portions of other foods might have scored equally well.)

The take-aways that were found wanting were: fried chicken and chips; cheeseburger and chips; fish in a bun; vegetarian pizza; fish and chips; baked potato with Cheddar cheese and butter; lamb samosas; sweet-and-sour pork with boiled rice.

There are doubtless other take-aways that fit with a healthy eating plan, and some of those that didn't do so well in the *Self Health* report could be made higher in fibre or lower in fat by altering their contents slightly: not having the chips; having the baked potato without butter, for example. But the research did show that it is possible to eat take-aways without breaking all your new resolutions for healthy eating.

Lunchboxes

Make wholemeal sandwiches with thick bread and a thin layer of spread. Home-made coleslaw with a low-fat mayonnaise, low-fat cheese, tinned fish, chicken and salad, or a savoury spread (peanut butter, for example) can all be used as fillings. Cold chicken, or wholemeal pastry quiche could be an occasional alternative to sandwiches. Natural yoghurts with fruit and nuts chopped up in them can be used for pudding. Sticks of celery, raw carrots, unsalted nuts and raisins, fruit and oatmeal biscuits all make good snack foods.

Public places – school dinners and hospitals

Cooking in British institutions has in the past been renowned for its lack of imagination and bland results. Overcooked and soggy vegetables, meat and fruit pies, custard and a bit of fish on a Friday are the memories of school dinners in the 1960s and 1970s. But things are beginning to change; combined pressure from consumers, dietitians and local authorities has resulted in significant improvements in the fare that is served in many public places.

In a survey of Local Education Authorities and schools, carried out for a *Which?* report on school dinners in September 1987, 88 per cent of LEAs and 68 per cent of schools claimed to be pursuing a 'healthy eating' policy. North Yorkshire LEA, for example, had created a character called 'Herbie', a carrot who encourages children to choose healthier foods from among the canteen-style meals available. Herbie proved so popular that there was a 23 per cent increase in the number of school lunches eaten. In most cases schools were running some classes on healthy eating, as well as providing more choice and variety in the dining-rooms. A look at the menus offered by a selection of schools supported the schools' claims – 75 per cent of the menus were judged by a nutritionist as at least offering the children the option of a healthy meal, although they could normally choose other foods as well.

A *Which?* report on hospital food in September 1988 found that Local Health Authorities were also making an attempt to improve the nutritional quality of the food served to patients, although they weren't doing as well as the schools. In a survey of hospitals, three-quarters of those who replied said they had a 'healthy eating' policy or were in the process of developing one. But although 60 per cent of the menus provided for the nutritionist to assess were thought to provide the option of choosing healthy meals, 40 per cent of the hospitals failed to reach an 'acceptable' score.

You're not alone

If you've decided to change your diet there are lots of things you can do on your own, by following the guidelines given here, but it is not always made as easy as it could be; there are some things that the Government and the food industry could do to make a would-be healthy eater's life easier. If full nutrition labelling were given on all foods, and claims for the nutrient content and 'naturalness' of food products were controlled in regulations, consumers trying to select foods as part of a healthy eating programmes would have a much easier time. But these sorts of legal changes need to be backed up by an information campaign, with posters and leaflets telling shoppers what the claims mean, how to use the nutrition labels and how to use new, alternative foods as part of a healthy eating programme.

There are also some existing regulations about food that could usefully be changed, for example, those relating to the farming of meat, that encourage the production of meat with a relatively high fat content, or the jam regulations that say jam must contain 66 grams of sugar in each 100 grams. These sorts of regulations hinder food manufacturers and farmers in any attempts they might otherwise make to produce the sort of food people need to follow a healthy eating programme.

Another problem is the fact that it can be more expensive to try to eat healthily. Since wholemeal flour, for example, is less processed than white, it is difficult to explain why it should cost more in the shops. In 1986 the London Food Commission calculated the amount it cost to buy 150 calories-worth of food of various different types. The 'healthier' alternative was not automatically more expensive, but was quite often, for example:

Low-fibre breakfast cereal   6.4p; high-fibre version   9.4p
White bread   3.4p; wholemeal bread   4.7p
Whole milk   9.3p; skimmed milk   18.4p
Mince   17.7p; lean beef   33p
Fatty pork   11.3p; lean pork   42.6p
Sausages   9.4p; poultry   34.7p
Canned fruit in syrup   18p; fresh fruit   30.8p.

One of the areas where people in the *Which?* dietary study had the greatest difficulty in changing their eating habits was snack foods; the fact is that it may be difficult to persuade yourself that an apple is going to be as rewarding as a chocolate bar, for example. There is a huge marketing opportunity for food manufacturers to capture by producing a wide range of snack foods that are consistent with healthy eating guidelines, but to date there is very little in the way of such foods on the shop shelves.

Food intake questionnaire: How much of these foods and their elements do you eat in a week?

(See page 126 for how to fill in the questionnaire)

Biscuits and cakes	Number of portions	Fat	Saturated fat	Salt	Added sugar	Fibre
Sweet biscuits (eg one chocolate covered or sandwich)	×	3 =	2 =	1 =	3 =	
Plain, sweet biscuits (eg one digestive or rich tea)	×	2 =	1 =	1 =	2 =	
Cake, plain or jam sponge (one slice – 50g)	×	3 =	1 =	3 =	18 =	
Cake or bun, rich (eg one slice gateau, butter-iced, chocolate, cream – 75g)	×	16 =	8 =	5 =	26 =	
Other cakes or buns (eg one slice Madeira, gingerbread, one rock cake, one doughnut or Danish pastry) – 75g	×	3 =	5 =	7 =	11 =	
Crispbread, one	×					1 =
		TOTAL	TOTAL	TOTAL	TOTAL	TOTAL

Dairy produce	Number of portions	Fat	Saturated fat	Salt	Added sugar	Fibre
Cheese, cream (eg Philadelphia) – 30g	[ ] ×	14 = [ ]	9 = [ ]			
Cheese, full-fat (eg Stilton, Cheddar) – 40g	[ ] ×	13 = [ ]	8 = [ ]			
Cheese, medium-fat (eg Edam, Camembert) – 40g	[ ] ×	9 = [ ]	6 = [ ]			
Cheese reduced fat (eg Shape & Tendale) – 40g	[ ] ×	6 = [ ]	4 = [ ]			
of which						
Cheese, high salt (eg blue, Camembert, processed and smoked) – 40g	[ ] ×			14 = [ ]		
Cheese, medium salt (eg Cheddar and other hard cheese, Edam) – 40g	[ ] ×			8 = [ ]		
Cheese, low salt (eg cottage, cream or curd) – 30g	[ ] ×			3 = [ ]		
Milk, whole (full-fat) – 140ml (¼ pint)	[ ] ×	5 = [ ]	3 = [ ]	1 = [ ]		

	Number of portions	Fat	Saturated fat	Salt	Added sugar	Fibre
Milk semi-skimmed – 140ml (¼ pint)	× [ ]	3 = [ ]	2 = [ ]	1 = [ ]		
Cream (one to two tablespoonfuls) – 45g	× [ ]	? = [ ]	10 = [ ]			
Yoghurt, full-fat, natural or fruit (eg Greek/Smetana) – one small pot	× [ ]	15 = [ ]	9 = [ ]	1 = [ ]		
Yoghurt, full-fat, natural or fruit (eg Greek/Smetana) – one small pot	× [ ]	2 = [ ]	1 = [ ]	1 = [ ]		
of which Yoghurt, fruit or flavoured – one small pot	× [ ]				22 = [ ]	
		TOTAL [ ]	TOTAL [ ]	TOTAL [ ]	TOTAL [ ]	TOTAL [ ]

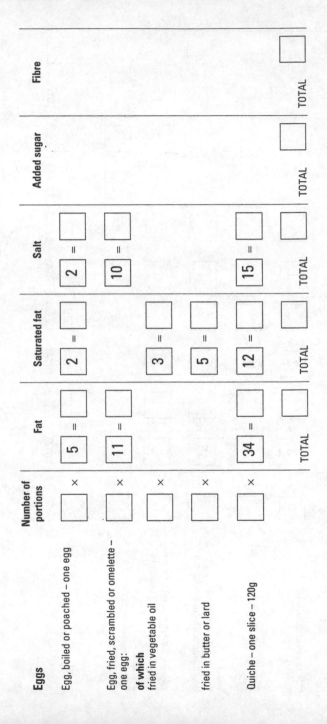

Eggs	Number of portions	Fat	Saturated fat	Salt	Added sugar	Fibre
Egg, boiled or poached – one egg	□ ×	5 = □	2 = □	2 = □		
Egg, fried, scrambled or omelette – one egg:	□ ×	11 = □		10 = □		
of which fried in vegetable oil	□ ×		3 = □			
fried in butter or lard	□ ×		5 = □			
Quiche – one slice – 120g	□ ×	34 = □	12 = □	15 = □		
		TOTAL □	TOTAL □	TOTAL □	TOTAL □	TOTAL □

Fat spread	Number of portions	Fat	Saturated fat	Salt	Added sugar	Fibre
Butter – 110g (¼lb)	× [ ]	91 = [ ]	59 = [ ]	25 = [ ]		
Low-fat margarine-type spread (eg Gold, Outline) – 110g (¼lb)	× [ ]	46 = [ ]	13 = [ ]	20 = [ ]		
Low-fat butter-type spread (eg Kerry Light) – 110g (¼lb)	× [ ]	46 = [ ]	29 = [ ]	20 = [ ]		
Margarine, high in polyunsaturates (eg sunflower, soya) – 110g (¼lb)	× [ ]	91 = [ ]	16 = [ ]	23 = [ ]		
Margarine, other soft – 110g (¼lb)	× [ ]	91 = [ ]	29 = [ ]	23 = [ ]		
Margarine, hard – 110g (¼lb)	× [ ]	91 = [ ]	40 . = [ ]	23 = [ ]		
		TOTAL [ ]	TOTAL [ ]	TOTAL [ ]	TOTAL [ ]	TOTAL [ ]

Meat and meat products	Number of portions		Fat		Saturated fat		Salt		Added sugar	Fibre
Bacon – 2 rashers	□	×	9	= □	4	= □	18	= □		
Ham – one slice	□	×	5	= □	2	= □	9	= □		
Liver sausage/pâté – one sandwich covering – 40g	□	×	7	= □	3	= □	6	= □		
Other processed meats (eg salami, tongue) – one slice	□	×	7	= □	3	= □	7	= □		
Tinned and processed meats (eg corned beef, spam or salami, tongue) – one slice	□	×	6	= □	2	= □	8	= □		
Beefburgers – one small – 35g	□	×	6	= □	3	= □	8	= □		
Sausages – one large – 60g	□	×	13	= □	5	= □	16	= □		
Meat pies, heavy (eg individual steak & kidney pie) – 200g	□	×	47	= □	19	= □	32	= □		

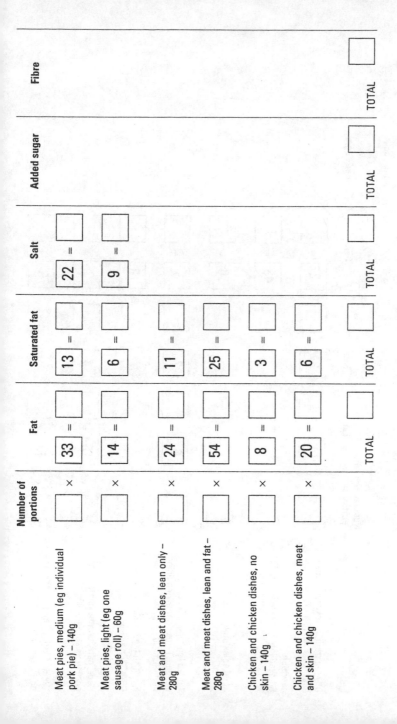

	Number of portions	Fat	Saturated fat	Salt	Added sugar	Fibre
Meat pies, medium (eg individual pork pie) – 140g	× [ ]	33 = [ ]	13 = [ ]	22 = [ ]		
Meat pies, light (eg one sausage roll) – 60g	× [ ]	14 = [ ]	6 = [ ]	9 = [ ]		
Meat and meat dishes, lean only – 280g	× [ ]	24 = [ ]	11 = [ ]			
Meat and meat dishes, lean and fat – 280g	× [ ]	54 = [ ]	25 = [ ]			
Chicken and chicken dishes, no skin – 140g	× [ ]	8 = [ ]	3 = [ ]			
Chicken and chicken dishes, meat and skin – 140g	× [ ]	20 = [ ]	6 = [ ]			
	TOTAL	[ ]	[ ]	[ ]	[ ]	[ ]
		TOTAL	TOTAL	TOTAL	TOTAL	TOTAL

Fish	Number of portions		Fat		Saturated fat		Salt		Added sugar	Fibre
Oily (eg trout, mackerel) – one average sized fish		×	14	=	3	=	2	=		
of which Smoked (eg mackerel) – one fish – 150g		×					43	=		
Smoked salmon – 60g		×					16	=		
Tinned (eg tuna, pilchards, sardines) – one sandwich filling portion – 50g		×	6	=	?	=	6	=		
Shellfish (eg cockles, mussels, prawns) – 40g		×					18	=		
Roes, pâté, taramosalata – one portion as starter – 40g		×	15	=	4	=	3	=		
White, fried (eg cod, haddock) – one steak or fillet – 110g		×	13	=			5	=		

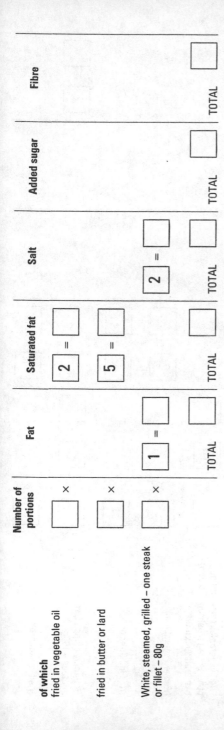

	Number of portions	Fat		Saturated fat		Salt		Added sugar	Fibre
of which fried in vegetable oil	☐ ×			2 = ☐					
fried in butter or lard	☐ ×			5 = ☐					
White, steamed, grilled – one steak or fillet – 80g	☐ ×	1 = ☐		☐		2 = ☐			
		☐ TOTAL		☐ TOTAL		☐ TOTAL		☐ TOTAL	☐ TOTAL

Vegetables: Fresh, frozen or tinned	Number of portions	Fat	Saturated fat	Salt	Added sugar	Fibre
Green leafy, fresh (eg cabbage, spinach, broccoli) – 90g	× ☐					3 = ☐
Peas, beans, lentils and chick peas – 90g	× ☐					9 = ☐
of which Tinned with added salt	× ☐			7 = ☐		
Fried vegetables (other than potatoes, eg mushroom, onion) – two tablespoonfuls:	× ☐	12 = ☐				
fried in vegetable oil	× ☐		2 = ☐			
fried in butter or lard	× ☐		7 = ☐			
Potatoes, chipped, roast, sautéed – 190g	× ☐	15 = ☐				2 = ☐
fried in vegetable oil	× ☐		2 = ☐			

fried in butter or lard □ ×

Potatoes, boiled or baked – 180g □ ×

Salad (eg mixed salad including tomatoes) – 110g □ ×

Root, fresh (eg carrots, parsnips) – 60g □ ×

Other tinned vegetables

Baked beans – half a small tin – 135g □ ×

Tomatoes – 100g □ ×

Sweetcorn – 90g □ ×

of which tinned with added salt – 90g □ ×

6 = □				3 = □
				1 = □
				2 = □
		16 = □		10 = □
				1 = □
		4 = □		5 = □
TOTAL □	TOTAL □	TOTAL □	TOTAL □	TOTAL □

Fruit: Fresh, frozen, stewed, or tinned in juice (unsweetened)

	Number of portions	Fat	Saturated fat	Salt	Added sugar	Fibre
Fruit (all types), tinned or stewed – 140g	☐ ×					1 = ☐
of which Sweetened	☐ ×				13 = ☐	
Avocado pear (half) – 75g	☐ ×	17 = ☐	2 = ☐			
Berries and fresh currants – 140g	☐ ×					4 = ☐
Apples, pears, bananas, citrus and other fruit (eg pineapple, grapes, melon, plums) – 100 – 200g	☐ ×					2 = ☐
Dried (apricots, prunes, sultanas, raisins) – 60g	☐ ×					10 = ☐
Yellow fruit (apricots, peach, mango, nectarine) – 100-150g	☐ ×					3 = ☐
		TOTAL ☐	TOTAL ☐	TOTAL ☐	TOTAL ☐	TOTAL ☐

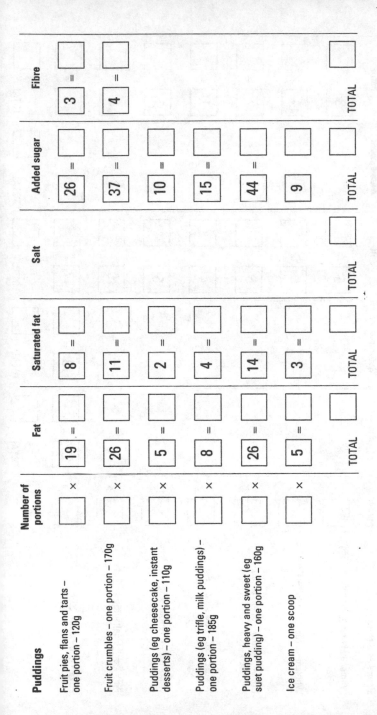

Puddings	Number of portions	Fat	Saturated fat	Salt	Added sugar	Fibre
Fruit pies, flans and tarts – one portion – 120g	☐ ×	19 = ☐	8 = ☐		26 = ☐	3 = ☐
Fruit crumbles – one portion – 170g	☐ ×	26 = ☐	11 = ☐		37 = ☐	4 = ☐
Puddings (eg cheesecake, instant desserts) – one portion – 110g	☐ ×	5 = ☐	2 = ☐		10 = ☐	
Puddings (eg trifle, milk puddings) – one portion – 185g	☐ ×	8 = ☐	4 = ☐		15 = ☐	
Puddings, heavy and sweet (eg suet pudding) – one portion – 160g	☐ ×	26 = ☐	14 = ☐		44 = ☐	
Ice cream – one scoop	☐ ×	5 = ☐	3 = ☐		9 ☐	
		TOTAL ☐	TOTAL ☐	TOTAL ☐	TOTAL ☐	TOTAL ☐

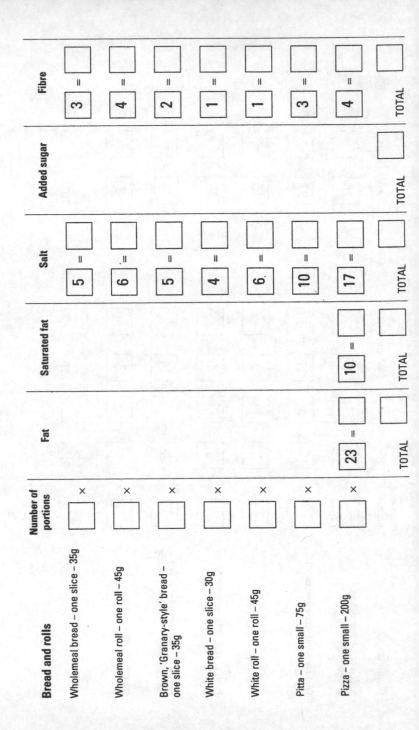

Bread and rolls	Number of portions	Fat	Saturated fat	Salt	Added sugar	Fibre
Wholemeal bread – one slice – 35g	×			5 =		3 =
Wholemeal roll – one roll – 45g	×			6 =		4 =
Brown, 'Granary-style' bread – one slice – 35g	×			5 =		2 =
White bread – one slice – 30g	×			4 =		1 =
White roll – one roll – 45g	×			6 =		1 =
Pitta – one small – 75g	×			10 =		3 =
Pizza – one small – 200g	×	23 =	10 =	17 =		4 =
		TOTAL	TOTAL	TOTAL	TOTAL	TOTAL

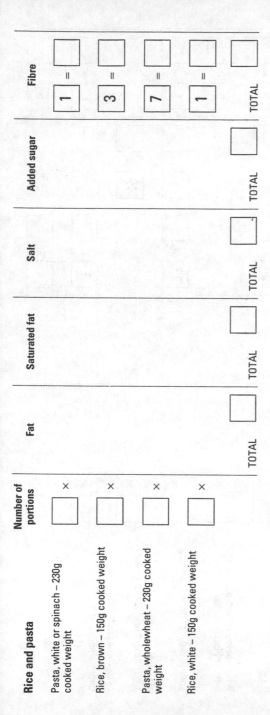

Breakfast cereals	Number of portions	Fat	Saturated fat	Salt	Added sugar	Fibre
High bran (eg All Bran, Bran Buds) – 50g	[ ] ×			13 = [ ]	9 = [ ]	14 = [ ]
Other bran-based (eg Bran Flakes) – 40g	[ ] ×			24 = [ ]	8 = [ ]	5 = [ ]
Wheat-based (flakes, puffs, two bisks or biscuits) – 40g	[ ] ×					5 = [ ]
Corn-based (eg Cornflakes) – 40g	[ ] ×			13 = [ ]	3 = [ ]	1 = [ ]
of which sugar-coated (eg Frosties) – 40g	[ ] ×				19 = [ ]	
Oats, porridge – 150g	[ ] ×			1 = [ ]		12 = [ ]
Muesli – 70g	[ ] ×			1 = [ ]		5 = [ ]

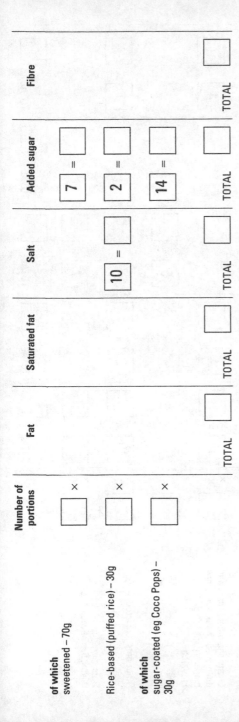

Number of portions	Fat	Saturated fat	Salt	Added sugar	Fibre
of which sweetened – 70g □ ×				7 = □	
Rice-based (puffed rice) – 30g □ ×			10 = □	2 = □	
of which sugar-coated (eg Coco Pops) – 30g □ ×				14 = □	
	TOTAL □	TOTAL □	TOTAL □	TOTAL □	TOTAL □

Snacks	Number of portions	Fat	Saturated fat	Salt	Added sugar	Fibre
Peanuts, one medium bag – 40g	□ ×	20 = □	4 = □	□		3 = □
of which Salted peanuts, one medium bag – 40g	□ ×			4 = □		
Crisps and other potato and cereal deep-fried snack foods, one medium pack – 35g **of which** salted	□ ×	13 = □	4 = □			4 = □
	□ ×			5 = □		
Other nuts (unsalted) – 40g	□ ×	19 = □	2 = □			1 = □
Olives, five olives – 15g	□ ×	1 = □		7 = □		
		□ TOTAL	□ TOTAL	□ TOTAL	□ TOTAL	□ TOTAL

Confectionery: Chocolate, toffee and chocolate-covered bars	Number of portions	Fat		Saturated fat		Salt	Added sugar		Fibre	
Large and heavy (eg Mars, Yorkie, Yorkie, Bounty, Fruit'n Nut) – 70g	☐ ×	17 =	☐	10 =	☐		39 =	☐		
Large and light (eg four-bar KitKat, Twix, Topic, Aero) – 50g	☐ ×	12 =	☐	7 =	☐		28 =	☐		
Small and light (eg Crunchy, Flake, Smarties, Treets, two-bar KitKat, Wispa, four chocolates or toffees) – 35g	☐ ×	8 =	☐	5 =	☐		20 =	☐		
Muesli bars – 30g	☐ ×	5 =	☐	1 =	☐		4 =	☐	4 =	☐
Sweets, boiled, mints, chews, pastilles and gums – one tube/pack – 35g	☐ ×						25 =	☐		
		TOTAL ☐		TOTAL ☐		TOTAL ☐	TOTAL ☐		TOTAL ☐	

Sugar and preserves

	Number of portions	Fat	Saturated fat	Salt	Added sugar	Fibre
Sugar, one teaspoonful – 5g	☐ ×				☐ = 5	
Jam, marmalade, honey and lemon curd, one slice bread-worth – 15g	☐ ×				☐ = 10	
		TOTAL ☐	TOTAL ☐	TOTAL ☐	TOTAL ☐	TOTAL ☐

Soft drinks (excluding low-calorie drinks)

	Number of portions	Fat	Saturated fat	Salt	Added sugar	Fibre
Cola, Lucozade, one small can – 200ml	☐ ×				☐ = 20	
Lemonade, squash (diluted), lime and blackcurrant cordials, and mixer drinks (eg tonics) one glass – 200ml	☐ ×				☐ = 11	
		TOTAL ☐	TOTAL ☐	TOTAL ☐	TOTAL ☐	TOTAL ☐

Sundries	Number of portions	Fat	Saturated fat	Salt	Added sugar	Fibre
Horlicks, Ovaltine, Drinking Chocolate – one mug	× □				12 = □	
Coffee whitener – one teaspoon	× □		3 = □			
Peanut butter – one slice bread-worth	× □	8 = □	2 = □	1 = □		
Soup, creamed, one small tin – 220g	× □	8 = □	2 = □	26 = □		
Salad dressings (eg mayonnaise or salad cream or french dressing) – 30g	× □	11 = □	2 = □	3 = □	3 = □	
Sauces/pickles (eg tomato, brown, Piccalilli), one teaspoon – 30g	× □			10 = □	3 = □	
		TOTAL □	TOTAL □	TOTAL □	TOTAL □	TOTAL □

Food intake questionnaire: How much of these foods and their elements do you eat in a week?

(See page 126 for how to fill in the questionnaire)

Biscuits and cakes	Number of portions		Fat		Saturated fat		Salt		Added sugar		Fibre
Sweet biscuits (eg one chocolate covered or sandwich)	☐	×	3	= ☐	2	= ☐	1	= ☐	3	= ☐	
Plain, sweet biscuits (eg one digestive or rich tea)	☐	×	2	= ☐	1	= ☐	1	= ☐	2	= ☐	
Cake, plain or jam sponge (one slice – 50g)	☐	×	3	= ☐	1	= ☐	3	= ☐	18	= ☐	
Cake or bun, rich (eg one slice gateau, butter-iced, chocolate, cream – 75g)	☐	×	16	= ☐	8	= ☐	5	= ☐	26	= ☐	
Other cakes or buns (eg one slice Madeira, gingerbread, one rock cake, one doughnut or Danish pastry) – 75g	☐	×	3	= ☐	5	= ☐	7	= ☐	11	= ☐	
Crispbread, one	☐	×									1 = ☐
			TOTAL ☐		TOTAL ☐		TOTAL ☐		TOTAL ☐		TOTAL ☐

Dairy produce	Number of portions	Fat		Saturated fat		Salt		Added sugar	Fibre
Cheese, cream (eg Philadelphia) – 30g	☐ ×	14 =	☐	9 =	☐				
Cheese, full-fat (eg Stilton, Cheddar) – 40g	☐ ×	13 =	☐	8 =	☐				
Cheese, medium-fat (eg Edam, Camembert) – 40g	☐ ×	9 =	☐	6 =	☐				
Cheese reduced fat (eg Shape & Tendale) – 40g	☐ ×	6 =	☐	4 =	☐				
of which Cheese, high salt (eg blue, Camembert, processed and smoked) – 40g	☐ ×					14 =	☐		
Cheese, medium salt (eg Cheddar and other hard cheese, Edam) – 40g	☐ ×					8 =	☐		
Cheese, low salt (eg cottage, cream or curd) – 30g	☐ ×					3 =	☐		
Milk, whole (full-fat) – 140ml (¼ pint)	☐ ×	5 =	☐	3 =	☐	1 =	☐		

	Number of portions	Fat	Saturated fat	Salt	Added sugar	Fibre
Milk semi-skimmed – 140ml (¼ pint)	× [ ]	3 = [ ]	2 = [ ]	1 = [ ]		
Cream (one to two tablespoonfuls) – 45g	× [ ]	? = [ ]	10 = [ ]			
Yoghurt, full-fat, natural or fruit (eg Greek/Smatana) – one small pot	× [ ]	15 = [ ]	9 = [ ]	1 = [ ]		
Yoghurt, full-fat, natural or fruit (eg Greek/Smetana) – one small pot	× [ ]	2 = [ ]	1 = [ ]	1 = [ ]		
of which Yoghurt, fruit or flavoured – one small pot	× [ ]				22 = [ ]	
		TOTAL [ ]	TOTAL [ ]	TOTAL [ ]	TOTAL [ ]	TOTAL [ ]

Eggs	Number of portions	Fat	Saturated fat	Salt	Added sugar	Fibre
Egg, boiled or poached – one egg	[ ] ×	5 = [ ]	2 = [ ]	2 = [ ]		
Egg, fried, scrambled or omelette – one egg:	[ ] ×	11 = [ ]		10 = [ ]		
of which fried in vegetable oil	[ ] ×		3 = [ ]			
fried in butter or lard	[ ] ×		5 = [ ]			
Quiche – one slice – 120g	[ ] ×	34 = [ ]	12 = [ ]	15 = [ ]		
		TOTAL [ ]	TOTAL [ ]	TOTAL [ ]	TOTAL [ ]	TOTAL [ ]

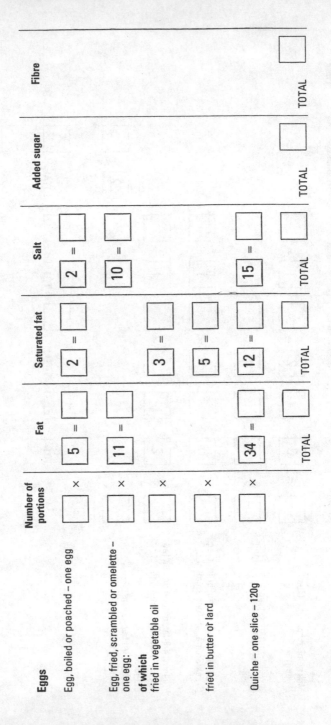

Fat spread	Number of portions		Fat		Saturated fat		Salt		Added sugar	Fibre
Butter – 110g (¼lb)	☐	×	91	= ☐	59	= ☐	25	= ☐		
Low-fat margarine-type spread (eg Gold, Outline) – 110g (¼lb)	☐	×	46	= ☐	13	= ☐	20	= ☐		
Low-fat butter-type spread (eg Kerry Light) – 110g (¼lb)	☐	×	46	= ☐	29	= ☐	20	= ☐		
Margarine, high in polyunsaturates (eg sunflower, soya) – 110g (¼lb)	☐	×	91	= ☐	16	= ☐	23	= ☐		
Margarine, other soft – 110g (¼lb)	☐	×	91	= ☐	29	= ☐	23	= ☐		
Margarine, hard – 110g (¼lb)	☐	×	91	= ☐	40	= ☐	23	= ☐		
				TOTAL ☐		TOTAL ☐		TOTAL ☐	TOTAL ☐	TOTAL ☐

Meat and meat products	Number of portions		Fat			Saturated fat			Salt			Added sugar	Fibre
Bacon – 2 rashers	☐	×	9	=	☐	4	=	☐	18	=	☐		
Ham – one slice	☐	×	5	=	☐	2	=	☐	9	=	☐		
Liver sausage/pâté – one sandwich covering – 40g	☐	×	7	=	☐	3	=	☐	6	=	☐		
Other processed meats (eg salami, tongue) – one slice	☐	×	7	=	☐	3	=	☐	7	=	☐		
Tinned and processed meats (eg corned beef, spam or salami, tongue) – one slice	☐	×	6	=	☐	2	=	☐	8	=	☐		
Beefburgers – one small – 35g	☐	×	6	=	☐	3	=	☐	8	=	☐		
Sausages – one large – 60g	☐	×	13	=	☐	5	=	☐	16	=	☐		
Meat pies, heavy (eg individual steak & kidney pie) – 200g	☐	×	47	=	☐	19	=	☐	32	=	☐		

	Number of portions	Fat	Saturated fat	Salt	Added sugar	Fibre
Meat pies, medium (eg individual pork pie) – 140g	☐ ×	33 = ☐	13 = ☐	22 = ☐		
Meat pies, light (eg one sausage roll) – 60g	☐ ×	14 = ☐	6 = ☐	9 = ☐		
Meat and meat dishes, lean only – 280g	☐ ×	24 = ☐	11 = ☐			
Meat and meat dishes, lean and fat – 280g	☐ ×	54 = ☐	25 = ☐			
Chicken and chicken dishes, no skin – 140g	☐ ×	8 = ☐	3 = ☐			
Chicken and chicken dishes, meat and skin – 140g	☐ ×	20 = ☐	6 = ☐			
		TOTAL ☐	TOTAL ☐	TOTAL ☐	TOTAL ☐	TOTAL ☐

Fish	Number of portions		Fat	Saturated fat	Salt	Added sugar	Fibre
Oily (eg trout, mackerel) – one average sized fish	☐	×	14 = ☐	3 = ☐	2 = ☐		
of which Smoked (eg mackerel) – one fish – 150g	☐	×			43 = ☐		
Smoked salmon – 60g	☐	×			16 = ☐		
Tinned (eg tuna, pilchards, sardines) – one sandwich filling portion – 50g	☐	×	6 = ☐	? = ☐	6 = ☐		
Shellfish (eg cockles, mussels, prawns) – 40g	☐	×			18 = ☐		
Roes, pâté, taramosalata – one portion as starter – 40g	☐	×	15 = ☐	4 = ☐	3 = ☐		
White, fried (eg cod, haddock) – one steak or fillet – 110g	☐	×	13 = ☐		5 = ☐		

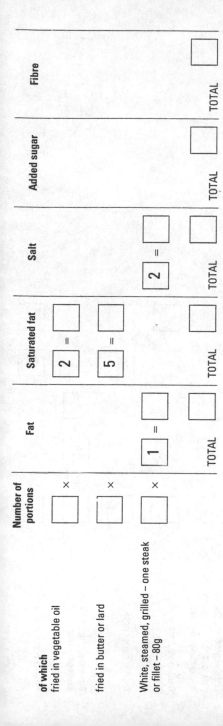

	Number of portions	Fat	Saturated fat	Salt	Added sugar	Fibre
of which fried in vegetable oil	☐ ×		2 = ☐			
fried in butter or lard	☐ ×		5 = ☐			
White, steamed, grilled – one steak or fillet – 80g	☐ ×	1 = ☐		2 = ☐		
		TOTAL ☐	TOTAL ☐	TOTAL ☐	TOTAL ☐	☐

Vegetables: Fresh, frozen or tinned

	Number of portions	Fat	Saturated fat	Salt	Added sugar	Fibre
Green leafy, fresh (eg cabbage, spinach, broccoli) – 90g	□ ×					3 = □
Peas, beans, lentils and chick peas – 90g	□ ×					9 = □
of which Tinned with added salt	□ ×			7 = □		
Fried vegetables (other than potatoes, eg mushroom, onion) – two tablespoonfuls:	□ ×	12 = □	2 = □			
fried in vegetable oil	□ ×					
fried in butter or lard	□ ×		7 = □			
Potatoes, chipped, roast, sautéed – 190g	□ ×	15 = □	2 = □			2 = □
fried in vegetable oil	□ ×					

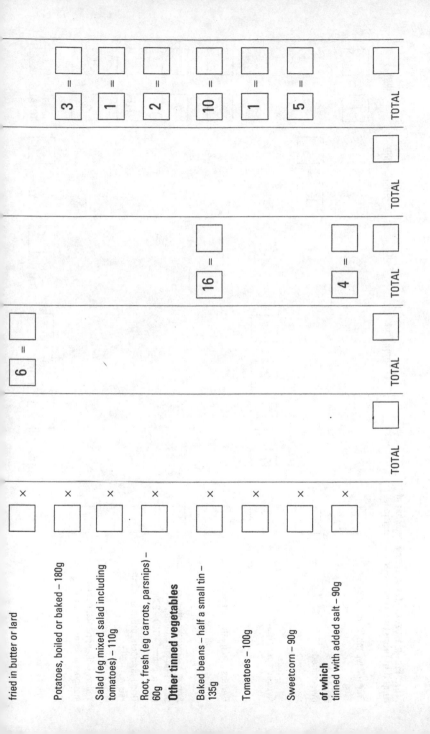

fried in butter or lard

Potatoes, boiled or baked – 180g

Salad (eg mixed salad including tomatoes) – 110g

Root, fresh (eg carrots, parsnips) – 60g

Other tinned vegetables

Baked beans – half a small tin – 135g

Tomatoes – 100g

Sweetcorn – 90g

of which tinned with added salt – 90g

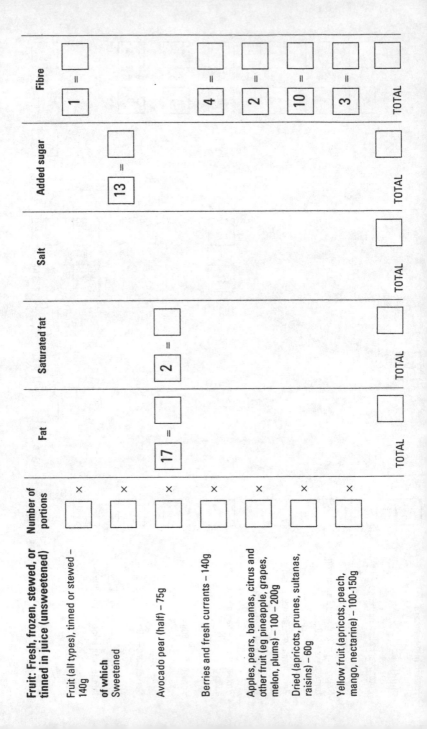

Fruit: Fresh, frozen, stewed, or tinned in juice (unsweetened)	Number of portions	Fat	Saturated fat	Salt	Added sugar	Fibre
Fruit (all types), tinned or stewed – 140g	☐ ×					1 = ☐
of which Sweetened	☐ ×				13 = ☐	
Avocado pear (half) – 75g	☐ ×	17 = ☐	2 = ☐			
Berries and fresh currants – 140g	☐ ×					4 = ☐
Apples, pears, bananas, citrus and other fruit (eg pineapple, grapes, melon, plums) – 100 – 200g	☐ ×					2 = ☐
Dried (apricots, prunes, sultanas, raisins) – 60g	☐ ×					10 = ☐
Yellow fruit (apricots, peach, mango, nectarine) – 100-150g	☐ ×					3 = ☐
		TOTAL ☐	TOTAL ☐	TOTAL ☐	TOTAL ☐	TOTAL ☐

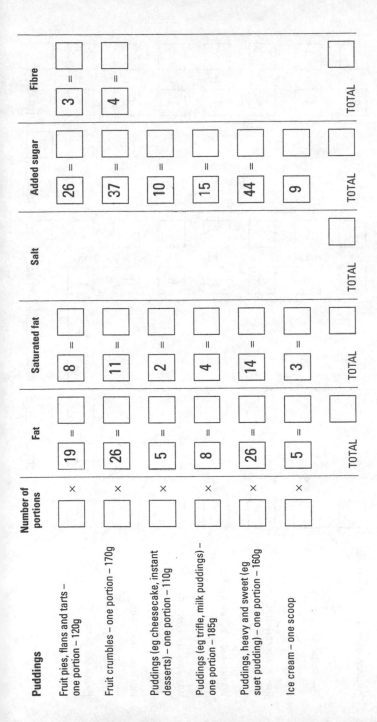

Puddings	Number of portions		Fat		Saturated fat		Salt	Added sugar		Fibre	
Fruit pies, flans and tarts – one portion – 120g		× [ ]	19 =	[ ]	8 =	[ ]		26 =	[ ]	3 =	[ ]
Fruit crumbles – one portion – 170g		× [ ]	26 =	[ ]	11 =	[ ]		37 =	[ ]	4 =	[ ]
Puddings (eg cheesecake, instant desserts) – one portion – 110g		× [ ]	5 =	[ ]	2 =	[ ]		10 =	[ ]		
Puddings (eg trifle, milk puddings) – one portion – 185g		× [ ]	8 =	[ ]	4 =	[ ]		15 =	[ ]		
Puddings, heavy and sweet (eg suet pudding) – one portion – 160g		× [ ]	26 =	[ ]	14 =	[ ]		44 =	[ ]		
Ice cream – one scoop		× [ ]	5 =	[ ]	3 =	[ ]		9	[ ]		
			TOTAL	[ ]	TOTAL	[ ]	TOTAL [ ]	TOTAL	[ ]	TOTAL	[ ]

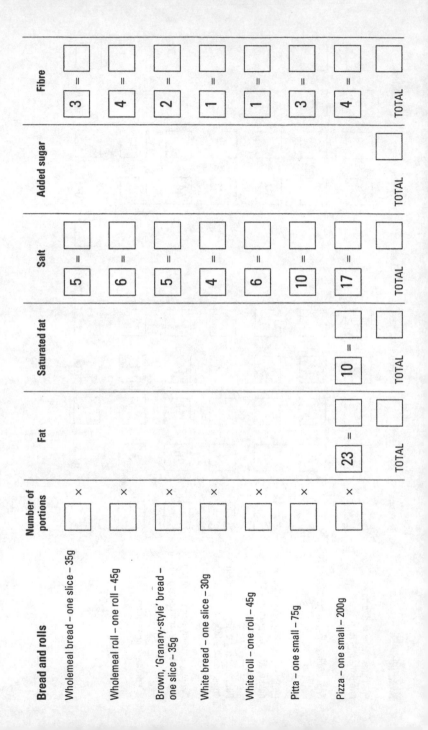

Bread and rolls	Number of portions	Fat	Saturated fat	Salt	Added sugar	Fibre
Wholemeal bread – one slice – 35g	☐ ×			5 = ☐		3 = ☐
Wholemeal roll – one roll – 45g	☐ ×			6 = ☐		4 = ☐
Brown, 'Granary-style' bread – one slice – 35g	☐ ×			5 = ☐		2 = ☐
White bread – one slice – 30g	☐ ×			4 = ☐		1 = ☐
White roll – one roll – 45g	☐ ×			6 = ☐		1 = ☐
Pitta – one small – 75g	☐ ×			10 = ☐		3 = ☐
Pizza – one small – 200g	☐ ×	23 = ☐	10 = ☐	17 = ☐		4 = ☐
		TOTAL ☐	TOTAL ☐	TOTAL ☐	TOTAL ☐	TOTAL ☐

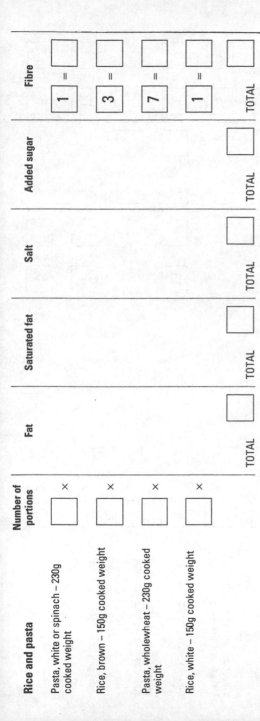

Rice and pasta	Number of portions		Fat	Saturated fat	Salt	Added sugar	Fibre	
Pasta, white or spinach – 230g cooked weight	☐	×					1 = ☐	
Rice, brown – 150g cooked weight	☐	×					3 = ☐	
Pasta, wholewheat – 230g cooked weight	☐	×					7 = ☐	
Rice, white – 150g cooked weight	☐	×					1 = ☐	
		TOTAL	☐	☐ TOTAL	☐ TOTAL	☐ TOTAL	☐ TOTAL	

Breakfast cereals	Number of portions	Fat	Saturated fat	Salt	Added sugar	Fibre
High bran (eg All Bran, Bran Buds) – 50g	☐ ×			13 = ☐	9 = ☐	14 = ☐
Other bran-based (eg Bran Flakes) – 40g	☐ ×			24 = ☐	8 = ☐	5 = ☐
Wheat-based (flakes, puffs, two bisks or biscuits) – 40g	☐ ×					5 = ☐
Corn-based (eg Cornflakes) – 40g	☐ ×			13 = ☐	3 = ☐	1 = ☐
of which sugar-coated (eg Frosties) – 40g	☐ ×				19 = ☐	
Oats, porridge – 150g	☐ ×			1 = ☐		12 = ☐
Muesli – 70g	☐ ×			1 = ☐		5 = ☐

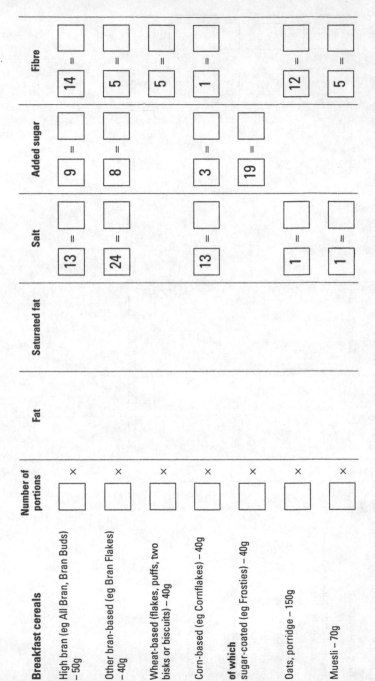

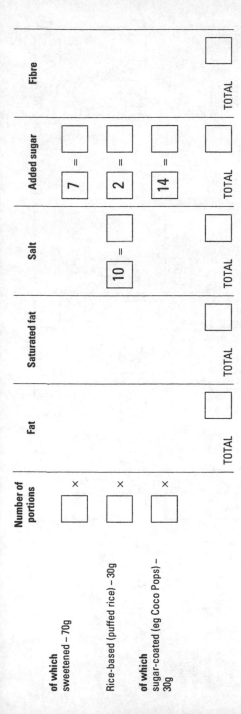

Number of portions		Fat	Saturated fat	Salt	Added sugar	Fibre
of which sweetened – 70g	☐ ×				7 = ☐	
Rice-based (puffed rice) – 30g	☐ ×			10 = ☐	2 = ☐	
of which sugar-coated (eg Coco Pops) – 30g	☐ ×				14 = ☐	
		☐ TOTAL	☐ TOTAL	☐ TOTAL	☐ TOTAL	☐

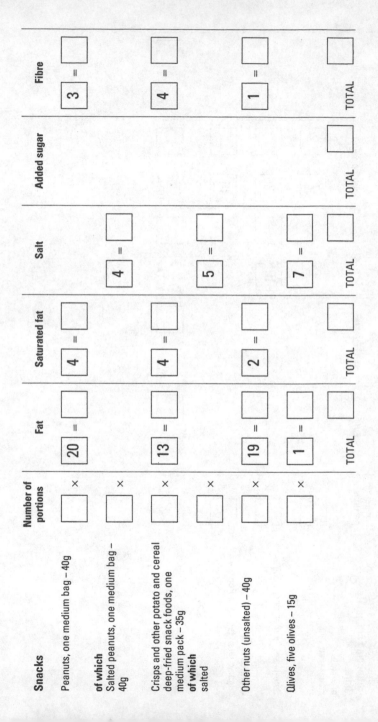

Snacks	Number of portions	Fat	Saturated fat	Salt	Added sugar	Fibre
Peanuts, one medium bag – 40g	× ☐	20 = ☐	4 = ☐			3 = ☐
of which Salted peanuts, one medium bag – 40g	× ☐			4 = ☐		
Crisps and other potato and cereal deep-fried snack foods, one medium pack – 35g **of which** salted	× ☐ × ☐	13 = ☐	4 = ☐	5 = ☐		4 = ☐
Other nuts (unsalted) – 40g	× ☐	19 = ☐	2 = ☐			1 = ☐
Olives, five olives – 15g	× ☐	1 = ☐		7 = ☐		
		TOTAL ☐	TOTAL ☐	TOTAL ☐	TOTAL ☐	TOTAL ☐

Confectionery: Chocolate, toffee and chocolate-covered bars	Number of portions	Fat	Saturated fat	Salt	Added sugar	Fibre
Large and heavy (eg Mars, Yorkie, Yorkie, Bounty, Fruit'n Nut) – 70g	[ ] ×	17 = [ ]	10 = [ ]		39 = [ ]	
Large and light (eg four-bar KitKat, Twix, Topic, Aero) – 50g	[ ] ×	12 = [ ]	7 = [ ]		28 = [ ]	
Small and light (eg Crunchy, Flake, Smarties, Treets, two-bar KitKat, Wispa, four chocolates or toffees) – 35g	[ ] ×	8 = [ ]	5 = [ ]		20 = [ ]	
Muesli bars – 30g	[ ] ×	5 = [ ]	1 = [ ]		4 = [ ]	4 = [ ]
Sweets, boiled, mints, chews, pastilles and gums – one tube/pack – 35g	[ ] ×			[ ]	25 = [ ]	
		TOTAL [ ]	TOTAL [ ]	TOTAL [ ]	TOTAL [ ]	TOTAL [ ]

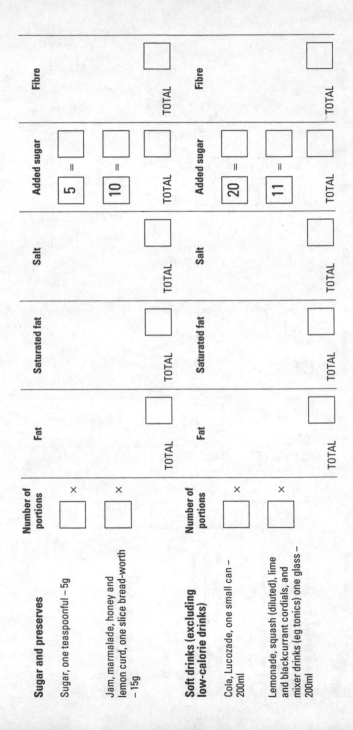

Sugar and preserves

	Number of portions	Fat	Saturated fat	Salt	Added sugar	Fibre
Sugar, one teaspoonful – 5g	☐ ×				☐ 5 = ☐	
Jam, marmalade, honey and lemon curd, one slice bread-worth – 15g	☐ ×				☐ 10 = ☐	
		TOTAL ☐	TOTAL ☐	TOTAL ☐	TOTAL ☐	TOTAL ☐

Soft drinks (excluding low-calorie drinks)

	Number of portions	Fat	Saturated fat	Salt	Added sugar	Fibre
Cola, Lucozade, one small can – 200ml	☐ ×				☐ 20 = ☐	
Lemonade, squash (diluted), lime and blackcurrant cordials, and mixer drinks (eg tonics) one glass – 200ml	☐ ×				☐ 11 = ☐	
		TOTAL ☐	TOTAL ☐	TOTAL ☐	TOTAL ☐	TOTAL ☐

Sundries	Number of portions	Fat	Saturated fat	Salt	Added sugar	Fibre
Horlicks, Ovaltine, Drinking Chocolate – one mug	☐ ×				12 = ☐	
Coffee whitener – one teaspoon	☐ ×	8 = ☐	3 = ☐	1 = ☐		
Peanut butter – one slice bread-worth	☐ ×	8 = ☐	2 = ☐	26 = ☐		
Soup, creamed, one small tin – 220g	☐ ×	11 = ☐	2 = ☐	3 = ☐		
Salad dressings (eg mayonnaise or salad cream or french dressing) – 30g	☐ ×	☐	2 = ☐	10 = ☐	3 = ☐	
Sauces/pickles (eg tomato, brown, Piccalilli), one teaspoon – 30g	☐ ×				3 = ☐	
		TOTAL ☐	TOTAL ☐	TOTAL ☐	TOTAL ☐	☐

Notes

Notes

Notes

Notes

Notes